Nestlé Nutrition Institute Workshop Series

Vol. 76

Limits of Human Endurance

Editors

Luc J.C. van Loon Maastricht, The Netherlands
Romain Meeusen Brussels, Belgium

KARGER

Nestlé
NutritionInstitute

Nestec Ltd., 55 Avenue Nestlé, CH–1800 Vevey (Switzerland)
S. Karger AG, P.O. Box, CH–4009 Basel (Switzerland) www.karger.com

Library of Congress Cataloging-in-Publication Data

Nestlé Nutrition Workshop (76th : 2012 : Oxford, England), author.
 Limits of human endurance / editors, Luc J.C. van Loon, Romain Meeusen.
    p. ; cm. -- (Nestlé Nutrition Institute workshop series, ISSN
1664-2147 ; vol. 76)
 Includes bibliographical references and index.
 ISBN 978-3-318-02408-1 (hbk. : alk. paper) -- ISBN 978-3-318-02409-8
(e-ISBN)
 I. Loon, Luc J. C. van, editor of compilation. II. Meeusen, Romain, editor
of compilation. III. Nestlé Nutrition Institute, issuing body. IV. Title. V.
Series: Nestlé Nutrition Institute workshop series ; v. 76. 1664-2147
 [DNLM: 1. Physical Endurance--physiology--Congresses. 2. Athletic
Performance--physiology--Congresses. 3. Exercise--physiology--Congresses.
4. Nutritional Physiological Phenomena--physiology--Congresses. W1 NE228D
v.76 2013 / QT 255]
 QP303
 612.7'6--dc23
                                                        2013018859

Printed on acid-free and non-aging paper (ISO 9706)
ISBN 978–3–318–02408–1
e-ISBN 978–3–318–02409–8
ISSN 1664–2147
e-ISSN 1664–2155

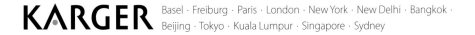

KARGER   Basel · Freiburg · Paris · London · New York · New Delhi · Bangkok ·
           Beijing · Tokyo · Kuala Lumpur · Singapore · Sydney

Contents

VII **Preface**

IX **Foreword**

XIII **Contributors**

1 **Caffeine, Exercise and the Brain**
Meeusen, R.; Roelands, B. (Belgium); Spriet, L.L. (Canada)

13 **Carnitine and Fat Oxidation**
Stephens, F.B.; Galloway, S.D.R. (UK)

25 **Hydration during Intense Exercise Training**
Maughan, R.J. (UK); Meyer, N.L. (USA)

39 **Intense Exercise Training and Immune Function**
Gleeson, M.; Williams, C. (UK)

51 **Physiological and Performance Adaptations to High-Intensity Interval Training**
Gibala, M.J. (Canada); Jones, A.M. (UK)

61 **Effect of β-Alanine Supplementation on High-Intensity Exercise Performance**
Harris, R.C. (UK); Stellingwerff, T. (Canada)

73 **Dietary Protein for Muscle Hypertrophy**
Tipton, K.D. (UK); Phillips, S.M. (Canada)

85 **The Role of Amino Acids in Skeletal Muscle Adaptation to Exercise**
Aguirre, N. (USA); van Loon, L.J.C. (The Netherlands); Baar, K. (USA)

103 **National Nutritional Programs for the 2012 London Olympic Games: A Systematic Approach by Three Different Countries**
Burke, L.M. (Australia); Meyer, N.L. (USA); Pearce, J. (UK)

121 **Concluding Remarks: Nutritional Strategies to Increase Performance Capacity**
van Loon, L.J.C. (The Netherlands); Meeusen, R. (Belgium)

127 **Subject Index**

For more information on related publications, please consult the NNI website:
www.nestlenutrition–institute.org

Preface

Nutrition is one of the key factors that modulate exercise performance. A healthy diet, adapted to the specific demands imposed upon by the individual athlete's training and competition, is required to allow optimal performance. Specific nutritional interventions have been developed to increase exercise endurance, allowing us to further improve sports performance in a variety of exercise tasks. In the 76th Nestlé Nutrition Institute Workshop, a group of expert scientists in the field of nutrition and exercise discussed the ergogenic properties of various nutritional interventions and presented research to show that dietary strategies can be applied to extend the limits of human endurance. Recent scientific findings on topics such as caffeine and its effect on the brain, carnitine and fat oxidation, ergogenic properties of β-alanine, dietary protein and muscle reconditioning, nutrition and immune status, and the importance of proper hydration were discussed. Last year, London hosted the 2012 Summer Olympics. Such an event provides a challenging landscape for nutritionists not only to ensure proper dietary management throughout the games but also to apply effective nutritional interventions that have been developed in the years preparing for the event. Success and failures of nutritional intervention were discussed from the perspective of 3 key nutritionists during the 2012 Olympics: Louise M. Burke for the Australian Institute of Sports, Nanna L. Meyer for the United States Olympic Committee, and Jeni Pearce for the English Institute of Sport. This workshop explored some of the many properties of dietary intervention to improve exercise performance capacity and, as such, to extend the limits of human endurance. We hope that the following chapters will provide the reader with many novel insights into the complex interaction between nutrition and exercise, allowing them to define more effective dietary strategies to improve health and performance.

Luc J.C. van Loon
Romain Meeusen

Foreword

The 76th Nestlé Nutrition Institute Workshop, The Olympic Sports Nutrition Conference, was timed to coincide with the London 2012 Olympic Games and was held in London and Oxford.

It brought together some of the world's greatest minds in sports nutrition to discuss and further our understanding of the ability of nutrition to support athletes in achieving the highest levels of performance and endurance.

Nutrition knowledge and practice has advanced since the last Olympic Games in Beijing, and the workshop gave the opportunity to examine emerging best practice in terms of eating plans, nutrition guidelines and hydration, alongside the latest discoveries such as the performance-enhancing effects and limitations of caffeine, carnitine, β-alanine and dietary protein.

Also discussed was the role of nutrition and supplements and the balance required to build specific performance capabilities, lower the risk of illness or injury and speed recovery rates.

While the focus of the conference was on elite athletes, it was interesting to note that some of these discoveries can be applied beyond this niche, to improve performance outcomes in the elderly for example.

We wish to warmly thank the chairpersons of this workshop Prof. Luc J.C. van Loon and Prof. Romain Meeusen for establishing an excellent scientific program.

We are also indebted to the renowned speakers and discussants that have furthered debate and understanding on this important topic through their presentations and participation. We thank the many experts who came for taking the time and effort to join us and discuss the influence nutrition can have on the limits of human endurance.

Finally, we wish to thank and congratulate Jeni Pearce from the English Institute of Sport, and her team, for their excellent logistical support and for exemplifying the best of British hospitality and helping us all to enjoy and embrace the Olympic spirit.

Eric Zaltas, MS, IOC Dipl. Sports Nutrition
Global Head R&D, Performance Nutrition
Nestlé Nutrition

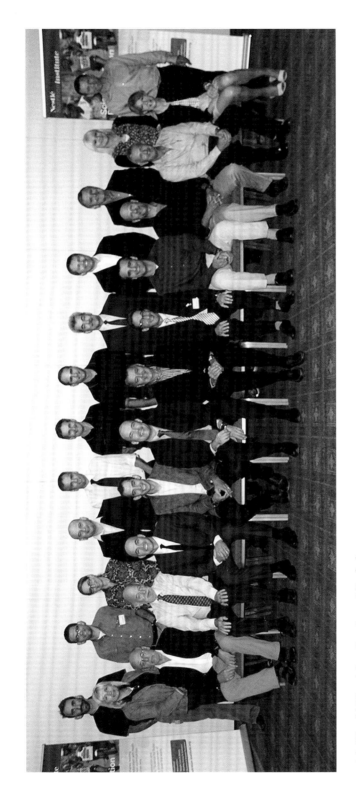

76th Nestlé Nutrition Institute Workshop
Oxford, August 15, 2012

.

Contributors

Chairpersons & Speakers

Prof. Luc J.C. van Loon
Department of Human Movement
Sciences
NUTRIM School for Nutrition, Toxicology
and Metabolism
Maastricht University Medical Centre+
NL–6200 MD Maastricht
The Netherlands
E-Mail L.vanLoon@
maastrichtuniversity.nl

Dr. Keith Baar
College of Biological Science
Dean's Office
University of California
Davis, One Shields Avenue
Davis, CA95616
USA
E-Mail fmblab@googlemail.com

Prof. Louise M. Burke
Australian Institute of Sport
Leverrier Crescent
Bruce, ACT 2616
Australia
E-Mail louise.burke@ausport.gov.au

Prof. Martin J. Gibala
Department of Kinesiology
McMaster University
1280 Main Street West
Hamilton, ON L8S 4K1
Canada
E-Mail gibalam@mcmaster.ca

Prof. Michael Gleeson
School of Sport, Exercise and Health
Sciences
Loughborough University
Ashby Road
Loughborough
Leicestershire LE11 3TU
UK
E-Mail m.gleeson@lboro.ac.uk

Prof. Roger C. Harris
Junipa Ltd.
4 Armstrong Close
Newmarket
Suffolk CB8 8HD
UK
E-Mail junipa@ymail.com

Prof. Ron J. Maughan
School of Sport, Exercise and Health
Sciences
Loughborough University
Ashby Road, Loughborough
Leicestershire LE11 3TU
UK
E-Mail R.J.Maughan@lboro.ac.uk

Prof. Romain Meeusen
Vrije Universiteit Brussel
Faculty LK
Dept. Human Physiology & Sports
Medicine
Pleinlaan 2
B-1050 Brussels
Belgium
E-Mail rmeeusen@vub.ac.be

Dr. Francis B. Stephens
MRC/Arthritis Research UK Centre for
Musculoskeletal Ageing Research
University of Nottingham Medical
School
Queen's Medical Centre
Nottingham NG7 2UH
UK
E-Mail francis.stephens@nottingham.
ac.uk

Prof. Kevin D. Tipton
Health and Exercise Sciences Research
Group
University of Stirling
Stirling, Scotland FK9 4LA
UK
E-Mail k.d.tipton@stir.ac.uk

Invited Discussants
Prof. Stuart M. Phillips/Canada
Prof. Lawrence L. Spriet/Canada
Dr. Trent Stellingwerff/Canada
Dr. Stuart D.R. Galloway/UK
Prof. Andrew M. Jones/UK
Dr. Jeni Pearce/UK
Dr. Clyde Williams/UK
Dr. Nanna L. Meyer/USA

Participant
Mr. Zibi Szlufcik/Germany

Nestlé Participants
Prof. Ferdinand Haschke/Switzerland
Dr. Natalia Wagemans/Switzerland
Mr. Frank Jimenez/USA
Mr. Eric Zaltas/USA

van Loon LJC, Meeusen R (eds): Limits of Human Endurance.
Nestlé Nutr Inst Workshop Ser, vol 76, pp 1–12, (DOI: 10.1159/000350223)
Nestec Ltd., Vevey/S. Karger AG., Basel, © 2013

Caffeine, Exercise and the Brain

Romain Meeusen[a] · Bart Roelands[a, b] · Lawrence L. Spriet[c]

[a]Department of Human Physiology and Sports Medicine, Vrije Universiteit Brussel, and
[b]Fund for Scientific Research Flanders, Brussels, Belgium; [c]Human Health and Nutritional
Sciences, University of Guelph, Guelph, ON, Canada

Abstract

Caffeine can improve exercise performance when it is ingested at moderate doses (3–6 mg/kg body mass). Caffeine also has an effect on the central nervous system (CNS), and it is now recognized that most of the performance-enhancing effect of caffeine is accomplished through the antagonism of the adenosine receptors, influencing the dopaminergic and other neurotransmitter systems. Adenosine and dopamine interact in the brain, and this might be one mechanism to explain how the important components of motivation (i.e. vigor, persistence and work output) and higher-order brain processes are involved in motor control. Caffeine maintains a higher dopamine concentration especially in those brain areas linked with 'attention'. Through this neurochemical interaction, caffeine improves sustained attention, vigilance, and reduces symptoms of fatigue. Other aspects that are localized in the CNS are a reduction in skeletal muscle pain and force sensation, leading to a reduction in perception of effort during exercise and therefore influencing the motivational factors to sustain effort during exercise. Because not all CNS aspects have been examined in detail, one should consider that a placebo effect may also be present. Overall, it appears that the performance-enhancing effects of caffeine reside in the brain, although more research is necessary to reveal the exact mechanisms through which the CNS effect is established. Copyright © 2013 Nestec Ltd., Vevey/S. Karger AG, Basel

Introduction

Caffeine can improve endurance performance when it is ingested at low–moderate dosages (3–6 mg/kg body mass); no further enhancement in performance is found when it is consumed at higher dosages (≥9 mg/kg) [1]. Caffeine supplementation is beneficial for sustained maximal endurance exercise, especially for time trial performance [1, 2]. Caffeine is also beneficial for high-intensity exercise, including team sports such as soccer and rugby, both of which are categorized by intermittent activity within a period of prolonged duration [3, 4]. The literature is equivocal when considering the effects of caffeine supplementation on strength-power performance, and additional research in this area is warranted [1, 5].

The effects of caffeine in reducing fatigue and increasing wakefulness and alertness have been recognized for a very long time. These properties have been targeted by shift workers, long-haul truck drivers, members of the military forces, athletes, and other populations who need to fight fatigue or prolong the capacity to undertake their occupational activities [2, 6, 7]. It has been shown that caffeine can enhance vigilance during bouts of extended exhaustive exercise, as well as periods of sustained sleep deprivation. The effects on attention, vigilance and alertness are established through the central nervous system (CNS), and several possible pathways and neurotransmitter systems are probable candidates for its action in the brain.

In this paper, we will discuss the possible mechanisms of how caffeine can influence performance through actions on the CNS.

How Does Caffeine Influence the Brain?

We are all aware of the fact that we need that morning cup of coffee, our daily dose of caffeine, to get started. We are more alert, more awake and feel better. Is this action really happening in the brain, or do we *think* caffeine works to keep us awake?

Caffeine is known to be a CNS stimulant, causing increased wakefulness, alertness, arousal, and vigilance as well as elevations of mood. Caffeine is quickly absorbed through the gastrointestinal tract. It is also lipid soluble and crosses the blood-brain barrier without difficulty.

Caffeine is an adenosine receptor antagonist, which means that it will influence the action of adenosine in a negative way [8]. The brain has a large number of adenosine receptors. The major known effect of adenosine is to decrease the concentration of many neurotransmitters, including serotonin, dopamine (DA), acetylcholine, norepinephrine, and glutamate. Caffeine blocks the adenosine receptors and opposes the effects of adenosine and therefore increases the concentration of these neurotransmitters in the CNS [8]. Increased actions of these neurotransmitters result in positive effects on vigilance, wakefulness, alertness, etc. [9].

Depending on the neurotransmitter system, caffeine can affect different brain areas with different functions. The most direct ways for caffeine to influ-

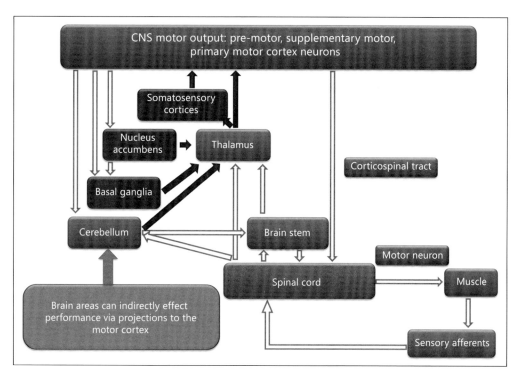

Fig. 1. Most direct ways for caffeine to effect muscular performance.

ence muscular performance is through its influence on the motor pathways (fig. 1). The CNS motor output originates from the pre-motor, supplementary motor and primary motor cortex neurons. The motor signal will travel through the corticospinal tract and the spinal cord to the muscle where contraction (exercise) takes place. A closed loop feedback system will create ascending signals through several possible pathways, influencing motor and other brain areas (fig. 1). Sensory afferents travel back via the spinal cord to the brain stem and the thalamus, which can be considered as the switch board for the afferent signals, and the cerebellum, which is important for motor function. From here, the signal travels to several key nuclei important in motor control such as the basal ganglia which are very rich in DA, the nucleus accumbens and the somatosensory cortices finally closing the feedback loop (fig. 1). All these brain areas can indirectly affect performance via projections to the motor cortex.

Several lines of evidence indicate that DA and adenosine systems interact in the brain. Both DA and adenosine have several receptor types; for DA the D_2 receptors and for adenosine the A_{2A} receptors play an important role in the stimulatory effect of caffeine. Striatal areas such as the neostriatum and nucleus accumbens are very rich in adenosine A_{2A} receptors, and there is a functional interface between striatal DA D_2 and adenosine A_{2A} receptors. This interaction has frequently been studied with regard to neostriatal motor functions. Nucleus accumbens DA is a critical component of the brain circuitry involved in behavioral activation and effort-related behavioral processes [10]. This means that both motor effects and motivational aspects will be influenced when adenosine receptors are blocked through caffeine, creating a greater dopaminergic drive.

This 'motor drive' effect was nicely shown by Davis et al. [11] who examined the effects of direct injections of caffeine into the brains of rats on their ability to run to exhaustion on a treadmill. In this controlled study, rats were injected with either vehicle (placebo), caffeine, an adenosine receptor agonist, or caffeine and the adenosine receptor agonist together. Rats ran 80 min in the placebo trial, 120 min after caffeine injection and only 25 min with adenosine receptor agonist. When caffeine and adenosine receptor agonist were given together, run time was not different from placebo. When the study was repeated with peripheral intraperitoneal injections instead of brain injections, there was no effect on run performance. The authors concluded that caffeine delayed fatigue through CNS effects, in part by blocking adenosine receptors [11].

But the influence of caffeine on exercise performance is not only situated in the 'pure' motor areas of the brain, as several other mechanisms can be responsible for the effect that caffeine may (or may not) have on exercise performance in humans.

DA and adenosine systems in the brain, possibly in nucleus accumbens, interact in the regulation of instrumental response output and effort-related choice behavior, probably because of the interaction between adenosine A_{2A} and DA D_2 receptors. This is likely related to the co-localization of these receptors on the same population of striatal and accumbens neurons. Characterization of the neurochemical mechanisms involved in regulating behavioral activation and effort-based choice behavior can shed light on these important facets of motivation, and also may serve to illustrate the relation between activational aspects of motivation (i.e. vigor, persistence and work output) and higher-order processes involved in motor control. Activational aspects of motivated behavior are highly adaptive because they enable organisms to surmount work-related response costs or obstacles that limit access to significant stimuli. This aspect is very important in sport performance because fatigue, effort and motivation are closely related in these specific brain areas.

The influence of caffeine on CNS functioning could be responsible for the positive effects on exercise performance. Some of these elements have been shown in experimental trials, while others still need further exploration.

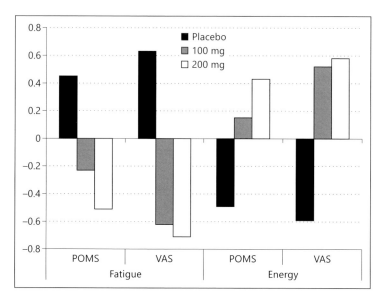

Fig. 2. Caffeine improves mood and performance and lowers the fatigue score in a dose-dependent manner. Both doses of caffeine produced uniform changes among measures of cognitive performance, the Visual Analogue Scale (VAS) mental energy measure and the Profile Of Mood State (POMS) vigor measure. Adapted from Maridakis et al. [12, 13].

Caffeine Improves Sustained Attention (Vigilance) and Reduces Symptoms of (Mental) Fatigue

Miridakis et al. [12, 13] conducted a double-blind, placebo-controlled experiment to compare the sensitivity to change of the cognitive performance and mood measures of mental energy following consumption of caffeine (100 and 200 mg). The authors defined 'mental energy' as the ability to perform mental tasks, the intensity of feelings of energy/fatigue, and the motivation to accomplish mental and physical tasks. Nine cognitive and five mood measures were used to quantify the effects of consuming 2 different doses of caffeine. As expected, caffeine attenuated the reduced feelings of energy and increased feelings of fatigue that occurred in the placebo condition. The sensitivity to 100 mg of caffeine was statistically different among the two energy measures, but not among the fatigue measures. The sensitivity to 200 mg of caffeine was statistically not different among the two energy or fatigue measures. Both doses of caffeine produced uniform changes among measures of cognitive performance, the Visual Analogue Scale mental energy measure and the Profile Of Mood State vigor measure (fig. 2). It seems that a small dose (100 mg) of caffeine is enough to produce small-to-moderate size improvements in stimulus response, improved target identification, and reductions in false alarms. Caffeine also improved mood and performance, and subjects scored better on a reaction time test and made fewer errors during the test.

The monoamines serotonin, DA and noradrenaline play a key role in signal transduction between neurons and exercise-induced changes in the concentrations of these neurotransmitters (especially serotonin and DA), and have been linked to central fatigue [9]. Although 'central fatigue' was originally linked with an increased serotonergic drive, Davis and Bailey [14] stated that not only increases in serotonin but an interaction between serotonin and DA would influence CNS fatigue, with a low ratio favoring improved performance and a high ratio decreasing motivation and augmenting lethargy and consequently decreasing performance.

Caffeine Reduces Skeletal Muscle Pain, Force Sensation and Perception of Effort during Exercise, and Increases Motivation to Sustain Effort

Moderate- to high-intensity exercise results in transient, naturally occurring muscle pain that is located in the activated musculature [15]. Caffeine is a non-selective adenosine antagonist with established anti-nociceptive actions. Muscle adenosine concentration is increased with muscle contractions [10], but whether adenosine plays a role in perceptions of naturally occurring skeletal muscle pain during exercise is unclear. The pain-reducing effect of blocking adenosine can be located both at the peripheral and central level, although the final perception and processing of the pain signal occurs through the CNS. Several studies have demonstrated that ingestion of caffeine significantly reduced muscle pain intensity ratings in males and females during 30 min of cycling on an ergometer at ~60% VO_{2peak} [15, 16] (fig. 3). In this study, caffeine doses of 5 and 10 mg/kg were used, and the ratings of perceived exertion (RPE) ratings were low in all trials. Several possible mechanisms exist for the caffeine-induced reduction in muscle pain during exercise. The hypoalgesia might stem from caffeine acting on peripheral or central adenosine receptors involved in the nociceptive system [17]. Alternatively, caffeine might indirectly influence the nociceptive system, for example, by altering muscle sensory processes. Separating the peripheral and central effects of caffeine in studies with humans is difficult, as caffeine has the potential to affect many tissues at once.

Also local muscle fatigue will be influenced by caffeine ingestion. Plaskett and Cafarelli [18] studied 15 subjects in a randomized, double-blind, repeated-

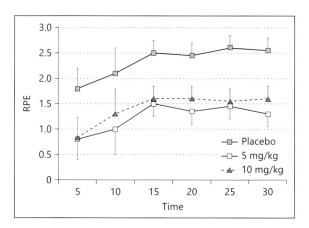

Fig. 3. Ingestion of caffeine significantly reduces muscle pain intensity ratings in males and females during 30 min of cycling on an ergometer at approximately 60% VO_{2peak} both in males and females. Adapted from Motl et al. [15, 16].

measures experiment to determine caffeine's ergogenic effects on neuromuscular variables that would contribute to increased endurance capacity. Subjects performed repeated submaximal isometric contractions (50% maximal voluntary contraction) of the right quadriceps to the limit of endurance 1 h after oral caffeine administration (6 mg/kg). Time to reach the limit of endurance increased by 17% after caffeine administration compared with the placebo trial. The results of this experiment showed that caffeine reduced force sensation during the first 10–20 s of the contraction. The rapidity of this effect suggests that caffeine exerts its effects neurally. The authors concluded that the caffeine-induced increase in performance may have been caused by a willingness to maintain near-maximal activation longer because of alterations in muscle sensory processes.

A consistent outcome of caffeine ingestion during exercise testing, regardless of mode, intensity, or duration of exercise, is an alteration in participants' perceptual response. This alteration has been manifested as either an increase in work output at a given RPE or effort sense or, more typically, a reduced RPE at a constant exercise intensity. Doherty and Smith [19] published a meta-analysis that clearly showed that the mean effect size for caffeine's influence on RPE during whole-body exercise is significantly greater than zero. In comparison to placebo, this effect represents almost a 6% reduction in the RPE during constant rate exercise. This evidence quantifies reports in the literature that caffeine has a noticeable effect on RPE.

This 'motivational' aspect of caffeine is probably through its stimulating effect on the dopaminergic system. It has been demonstrated that a moderate dose of the DA stimulant D-amphetamine increases willingness to exert effort in healthy young adults, particularly when reward probability is low. Adenosine receptors interact with DA receptors to influence both the reinforcing effects of psychostimulants and effort exerted for rewards.

Caffeine Increases Tremor

Accuracy is important in most sports, but it is known that 'overinfluencing' the motor areas of the brain might have negative effects. Fine motor skills are important in several sports and especially sports that combine these features with endurance exercise (e.g. biathlon and all the stop and go sports like football, ice and field hockey, basketball). Any overinfluencing side effects can negatively affect performance. Miller et al. [20] examined the effects of a single oral dose of caffeine at typical daily levels of consumption (1 and 3 mg caffeine/kg body mass). They found a significant increase in tremor compared to placebo at 3 but not 1 mg caffeine/kg. Although many studies have recently reported significant effects of caffeine on various cognitive and psychomotor tasks, fewer studies have reported the direct effects of caffeine on physiological tremor. This effect does not have a real importance in endurance sports; however, in sports where accuracy (biathlon, shooting, archery, basketball, etc.) plays a role, this CNS side effect of caffeine should be avoided.

Caffeine Can Have a Placebo Effect

It has also been suggested that beliefs about the effects of caffeine or caffeine expectancies may factor into the performance effects of caffeine. The effects of caffeine dose and/or caffeine instructions on performance (e.g. reaction time) or subjective outcomes (e.g. arousal) are more pronounced among participants who hold expectancies that caffeine produces those effects. This was nicely shown in a study from Harrel and Juliano [21]. After overnight caffeine abstinence, participants were given coffee and were told either that caffeine would enhance or impair performance. This was crossed with the consumption of a placebo drink. Relative to placebo, caffeine improved reaction time and accuracy on the rapid visual information processing task, a measure of vigilance. However, among participants given placebo coffee, the 'impair' instructions produced better performance than the 'enhance' instructions. Caffeine also improved psychomotor performance as indicated by a finger tapping task with no

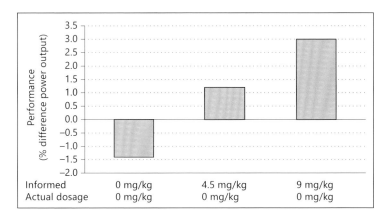

Fig. 4. Caffeine can have a placebo effect. Subjects performed a 10-km time trial and were informed to receive a placebo, 4.5 mg/kg caffeine, and 9.0 mg/kg caffeine, randomly assigned. However, placebos were administered in all experimental conditions. Adapted from Harrell and Juliano [21].

main effects of expectancy or interactions. These results provide evidence that subjective and behavioral outcomes of drug use at rest are influenced by the expected effects of drug.

Beedie et al. [22] showed that the placebo effect could also play an important role in the possible performance-enhancing effects of caffeine during exercise. The placebo effect – a change attributable only to an individual's belief in the efficacy of a treatment – might provide a worthwhile improvement in physical performance. The authors explored the placebo effect in laboratory cycling performance using quantitative and qualitative methods. Six well-trained male cyclists undertook two baseline and three experimental 10-km time trials. Subjects were informed that in the experimental trials they would each receive a placebo, 4.5 mg/kg caffeine, and 9.0 mg/kg caffeine, randomly assigned. However, placebos were administered in all experimental conditions (fig. 4).

Surprisingly, a dose-response relationship was evident in experimental trials, with subjects producing 1.4% less power than at baseline when they believed they had ingested a placebo, 1.3% more power than at baseline when they believed they had ingested 4.5 mg/kg caffeine, and 3.1% more power than at baseline when they believed they had ingested 9.0 mg/kg caffeine. This study clearly showed that placebo effects are associated with the administration of caffeine and that these effects may directly or indirectly enhance performance in well-trained cyclists. Although these results seem to be very convincing, several points need to be raised about this experiment. There were only 6 subjects, there were no actual caffeine trials to see how large any caffeine-induced performance increases would have been, and the exercise task – a 10 km time trial – would have lasted well under 20 min for well-trained cyclists – so quite short for caffeine-induced effects.

Caffeine and Exercise Performance in Different Ambient Conditions

Exercise capacity is enhanced after caffeine ingestion. It was originally proposed that caffeine mobilized free fatty acids from adipose tissue, resulting in higher rates of fat oxidation and sparing of muscle glycogen. More recently, this so-called 'metabolic' theory has been dismissed as a universal explanation for the ergogenic effect of caffeine on endurance exercise performance, and it seems that caffeine exerts its effect via central fatigue mechanisms or by facilitating muscle function. Caffeine has been shown to exert its ergogenic effects in normal ambient temperature. However, only a few studies examined the effects of adenosine receptor antagonism at high environmental temperatures. Most studies found increased core temperatures during exercise, non-attributable to metabolic heat production, as subjects did not push higher power outputs, but probably related to the influence of caffeine on the adenosine receptors and consequently DA concentration. The results on performance were divergent, with some studies showing improvements in time trial performance with caffeine ingestion [23, 24], while other studies showed that caffeine did not alter exercise performance on a preloaded time trial [25, 26]. Ganio et al. [23] showed that caffeine attenuated the perception of effort while exercising at 33°C, as was already reported at normal ambient temperature. They also found that, although caffeine improved exercise capacity, its effect on leg muscle pain was dependent on ambient temperature. Although exercise in the heat increases muscle pain compared to a cooler environment, caffeine reduced this pain [24]. Although more research is necessary to confirm these studies, it is clear that environmental conditions play an important role in the exertion of effects mediated by caffeine.

Conclusion

There is an extensive amount of scientific literature associated with caffeine supplementation. It is evident that caffeine is ergogenic for sport performance. It is now believed that most of the ergogenic effect of caffeine resides in the brain. Caffeine is an antagonist of the adenosine receptors and will therefore increase several neurotransmitter concentrations in the brain. One candidate mechanism for this performance-enhancing effect is the influence on the dopaminergic system, by maintaining the dopaminergic drive, which is very important for motivation, sustained attention and motor drive.

Disclosure Statement

The authors of this chapter do not have any relationship to disclose.

References

1 Goldstein R, Ziegenfuss T, Kalman D, et al: International society of sports nutrition position stand: caffeine and performance. J Intern Soc Sports Nutr 2010;7:5.
2 Burke L: Caffeine and sport performance. Appl Physiol Nutr Metab 2008;33:1319–1334.
3 Gant N, Ali A, Foskett A: The influence of caffeine and carbohydrate coingestion on simulated soccer performance. Int J Sports Nutr Exerc Metab 2010;20:191–197.
4 Roberts SP, Stokes KA, Trewartha G, et al: Effects of carbohydrate and caffeine ingestion on performance during a rugby union simulation protocol. J Sports Sci 2010;28:833–842.
5 Warren G, Park N, Maresca R, et al: Effect of caffeine ingestion on muscular strength and endurance: a meta-analysis. Med Sci Sports Exerc 2010;42:1375–1387.
6 Lieberman HR, Wurtman RJ, Emde GG, et al: The effects of low doses of caffeine on human performance and mood. Psychopharmacology 1987;92:308–312.
7 Olson, CA, Thornton JA, Adam GE, et al: Effects of 2 adenosine antagonists, quercetin and caffeine, on vigilance and mood. J Clin Psychopharmacol 2010;30:573–578.
8 Fredholm B: Adenosine, adenosine receptors and the actions of caffeine. Pharmacol Toxicol 1995;76:93–101.
9 Meeusen R, Watson P, Hasegawa H, et al: Central fatigue: the serotonin hypothesis and beyond. Sports Med 2006;36:881–909.
10 Salamone J, Farrar A, Font L, et al: Differential actions of adenosine A1 and A2A antagonists on the effort-related effects of dopamine D2 antagonism. Behav Brain Res 2009;201:216–222.
11 Davis J, Zhao Z, Stock H, et al: Central nervous system effects of caffeine and adenosine on fatigue. Am J Physiol Regul Integr Comp Physiol 2003;284:R399–R404.
12 Maridakis V, O'Connor P, Tomporowski P: Sensitivity to change in cognitive performance and mood measures of energy and fatigue in response to morning caffeine alone or in combination with carbohydrate. Int J Neurosci 2009;119:1239–1258.
13 Maridakis V, Herring M, O'Connor P: Sensitivity to change in cognitive performance and mood measures of energy and fatigue in response to differing doses of caffeine or breakfast. Int J Neurosci 2009;119:975–994.
14 Davis JM, Bailey SP: Possible mechanisms of central nervous system fatigue during exercise. Med Sci Sports Exerc 1997;29:45–57.
15 Motl R, O'Connor P, Dishman R: Effect of caffeine on perceptions of leg muscle pain during moderate intensity cycling exercise. J Pain 2003;4:316–321.
16 Motl R, O'Connor P, Tubandt L, et al: Effect of caffeine on leg muscle pain during cycling exercise among females. Med Sci Sports Exerc 2006;38:598–604.
17 Sawynok J, Liu X: Adenosine in the spinal cord and periphery: release and regulation of pain. Prog Neurobiol 2003;69:313–340.
18 Plaskett C, Cafarelli E: Caffeine increases endurance and attenuates force sensation during submaximal isometric contractions. J Appl Physiol 2001;91:1535–1544.
19 Doherty M, Smith P: Effects of caffeine ingestion on rating of perceived exertion during and after exercise: a meta-analysis. Scand J Med Sci Sports 2005;15:69–78.

20 Miller L, Lombardo T, Fowler S: Caffeine, but not time of day, increases whole-arm physiological tremor in non-smoking moderate users. Clin Exp Pharmacol Physiol 1998;25: 131–133.

21 Harrell P, Juliano L: Caffeine expectancies influence the subjective and behavioral effects of caffeine. Psychopharmacology 2009;207: 335–342.

22 Beedie C, Stuart E, Coleman D, et al: Placebo effects of caffeine on cycling performance. Med Sci Sports Exerc 2006;38:2159–2164.

23 Ganio M, Johnson E, Klau J, et al: Effect of ambient temperature on caffeine ergogenicity during endurance exercise. Eur J Appl Physiol 2011;111:1135–1146.

24 Ganio M, Johnson E, Lopez R, et al: Caffeine lowers muscle pain during exercise in hot but not cool environments. Physiol Behav 2011; 102:429–435.

25 Cheuvront S, Ely B, Kenefick R, et al: No effect of nutritional adenosine receptor agonists on exercise performance in the heat. Am J Physiol Regul Integr Comp Physiol 2009; 296:R394–R401.

26 Roelands B, Buyse L, Pauwels F, et al: No effect of caffeine on exercise performance in high ambient temperature. Eur J Appl Physiol 2011;111:3089–3095.

van Loon LJC, Meeusen R (eds): Limits of Human Endurance.
Nestlé Nutr Inst Workshop Ser, vol 76, pp 13–23, (DOI: 10.1159/000350224)
Nestec Ltd., Vevey/S. Karger AG., Basel, © 2013

Carnitine and Fat Oxidation

Francis B. Stephens[a] · Stuart D.R. Galloway[b]

[a] MRC/Arthritis Research UK Centre for Musculoskeletal Ageing Research,
University of Nottingham Medical School, Queen's Medical Centre, Nottingham,
[b] School of Sport, University of Stirling, Stirling, UK

Abstract

Fat and carbohydrate are the primary fuel sources for mitochondrial ATP production in human skeletal muscle during endurance exercise. However, fat exhibits a relatively low maximal rate of oxidation in vivo, which begins to decline at around 65% of maximal oxygen consumption (VO_2max) when muscle glycogen becomes the major fuel. It is thought that if the rate of fat oxidation during endurance exercise could be augmented, then muscle glycogen depletion could be delayed and endurance improved. The purpose of the present review is to outline the role of carnitine in skeletal muscle fat oxidation and how this is influenced by the role of carnitine in muscle carbohydrate oxidation. Specifically, it will propose a novel hypothesis outlining how muscle free carnitine availability is limiting to the rate of fat oxidation. The review will also highlight recent research demonstrating that increasing the muscle carnitine pool in humans can have a significant impact upon both fat and carbohydrate metabolism during endurance exercise which is dependent upon the intensity of exercise performed.   Copyright © 2013 Nestec Ltd., Vevey/S. Karger AG, Basel

Introduction

Fat and carbohydrate are the primary fuel sources for mitochondrial ATP production in human skeletal muscle during endurance exercise. Fat constitutes the largest energy reserve in the body, and in terms of the amount available it is not limiting to endurance exercise performance. However, fat exhibits a relatively low maximal rate of oxidation in vivo, which begins to decline at around 65% of maximal oxygen consumption (VO_2max) when muscle glycogen becomes the major fuel supporting ATP homeostasis [1–3]. The muscle glycogen stores are limited, and it has been well established that muscle glycogen deple-tion coincides with fatigue during high-intensity endurance exercise [4]. As fa-tigue can be postponed by increasing pre-exercise muscle glycogen content [4], it is thought that augmenting the rate of fat oxidation during endurance exercise could delay glycogen depletion and improve endurance exercise performance. Indeed, it has long been known that enhanced fat oxidation is one of the main muscle adaptations to endurance exercise training [5]. For this reason, a large amount of research towards the end of the 20th century was directed towards investigating the effects of L-carnitine supplementation on endurance exercise performance as carnitine is known to play an essential role in the translocation of fat into the mitochondria, which is considered to be a key rate-limiting step in fat oxidation [6]. However, scientific interest in L-carnitine as an ergogenic aid soon declined when it became apparent that L-carnitine feeding did not alter fat oxidation, exercise performance or, more importantly, impact upon the muscle carnitine pool in humans. The purpose of the present review is to out-line the role of carnitine in skeletal muscle fat oxidation and how this is influ-enced by the role of carnitine in carbohydrate oxidation, and to highlight more recent research demonstrating that the muscle carnitine pool can indeed be in-creased in humans and have a significant impact on these roles during endur-ance exercise.

Role of Carnitine in Skeletal Muscle Fat Oxidation

Irving Fritz and colleagues first established that mitochondria in a variety of tis-sues are impermeable to fatty acyl-CoA, but not to fatty acylcarnitine, and that carnitine and carnitine palmitoyltransferase (CPT) are essential for the translo-cation of long-chain fatty acids into skeletal muscle mitochondria for β-oxidation [e.g. 7]. Since these discoveries, it has been established that CPT1, situated with-in the outer mitochondrial membrane, catalyzes the reversible esterification of carnitine with long-chain acyl-CoA to form long-chain acylcarnitine. Cytosolic acylcarnitine is then transported into the mitochondrial matrix in a simultane-ous 1:1 exchange with intramitochondrial free carnitine via the carnitine acyl-carnitine translocase (CACT), which is situated within the mitochondrial inner membrane. Once inside the mitochondrial matrix, acylcarnitine is transesteri-fied back to free carnitine and long-chain acyl-CoA in a reaction catalyzed by CPT2, which is situated on the matrix side of the inner mitochondrial mem-brane (see fig. 1). The intramitochondrial long-chain acyl-CoA is then oxidized and cleaved by the β-oxidation pathway. The significance of this 'carnitine cycle' to fat oxidation during exercise is highlighted in patients with carnitine, CPT2,

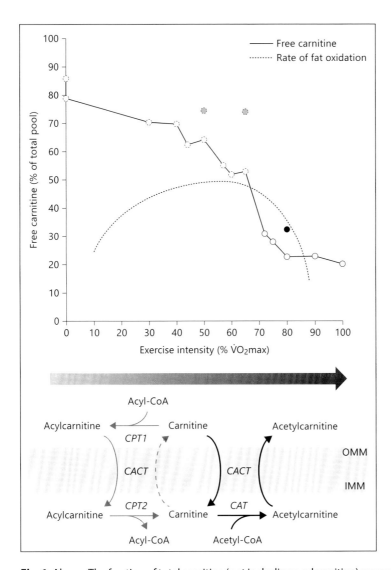

Fig. 1. Above: The fraction of total carnitine (not including acylcarnitine) represented as free carnitine in human vastus lateralis muscle at rest and following 4–30 min of exercise on a cycle ergometer at various exercise intensities in relation to the rate of fat oxidation. Open circles are a review of results taken from references [2, 17, 19–22, 24] under standard conditions. Closed circles are results from references [17, 24] after the muscle free carnitine pool has been manipulated by 6 months of L-carnitine and carbohydrate feeding [24] or at 65% VO_2max by reducing glycolytic flux [17]; these interventions shift the rate of fat oxidation curve up, rather than to the right. Below: Schematic diagram of the dual metabolic role of free carnitine within skeletal muscle fat (grey arrows) and carbohydrate (black arrows) oxidation. The small intramitochondrial free carnitine pool is delivered to the catalytic site of CPT1 in a 1:1 exchange with acylcarnitine produced from the CPT1 reaction, and is hypothetically limiting to CPT1. Excess acetyl-CoA from the PDC reaction is buffered by the large extramitochondrial free carnitine pool via the CAT reaction, which 'steals' intramitochondrial free carnitine with increasing exercise intensity (arrow). OMM = Outer mitochondrial membrane; IMM = inner mitochondrial membrane.

or CACT deficiency (CPT1 deficiency appears to be incompatible with life) who typically experience severely reduced rates of fat oxidation during prolonged exercise along with muscle pain and weakness, hypoglycemia, and hypoketosis. For a detailed review of this fat translocation process, see McGarry and Brown [8].

CPT1 is considered to be the rate-limiting enzyme for long-chain fatty acid entry into the mitochondria and oxidation, but carnitine is not thought to be rate limiting to CPT1. Indeed, the concentration of carnitine in skeletal muscle is around 5 mM intracellular water [9] and far in excess of the in vitro Michaelis-Menten constant (K_m) of muscle CPT1 for carnitine of approximately 0.5 mM [6]. However, the enzymes of the carnitine cycle co-immunoprecipitate and are mainly located in the specialized contact sites between outer- and inner-mitochondrial membranes in order to allow metabolic channeling [10]. Thus, it is the premise of the present chapter that the intramitochondrial content of free carnitine determines carnitine availability to CPT1 and, as this is around 10% of the whole muscle carnitine pool [11], that carnitine could be rate limiting to the CPT1 reaction. By way of example, translocation of acylcarnitine from the CPT1 reaction into the mitochondrial matrix in order to allow continuation of the CPT1 reaction (acylcarnitine is a potent inhibitor of CPT1 flux) is dependent upon exchange with intramitochondrial free carnitine to the CPT1 catalytic site via CACT. It stands to reason, therefore, that any change in the intramitochondrial free carnitine pool will likely impact upon CPT1 flux, which may partly explain how the rate of fat oxidation is regulated.

Regulation of the Rate of Skeletal Muscle Fat Oxidation

While CPT1 is considered a key site in the regulation of the rate of fat oxidation, it must be noted that there are several other potential control points that could influence the decline in the rate of fat oxidation in skeletal muscle during high-intensity endurance exercise. These other control points include: (1) regulation of lipolysis within adipose tissue and intramuscular triacylglycerol pools; (2) transport and delivery of circulating free fatty acids from adipose tissue stores to working skeletal muscle; (3) transport of fatty acids across the muscle cell membrane and within the cell cytosol to the outer mitochondrial membrane, and (4) intramitochondrial enzymatic reactions distal to CPT1. The contribution of each of these control points to the regulation of fat oxidation within contracting skeletal muscle is not yet fully understood, but it is likely that the role of each of these will vary depending upon the intensity of exercise and will likely all respond to exercise training.

The enzymes in adipose tissue and skeletal muscle that mobilize free fatty acids from triacylglycerol stores are known to be stimulated by epinephrine, norepinephrine, adenosine and some peptides, and are inhibited by insulin, and thus impaired mobilization would seem unlikely to be a limiting factor at exercise intensities above 65% of VO_2max. However, the release of mobilized fatty acids from adipose tissue into the circulation could be limiting if adipose tissue blood flow was compromised at higher exercise intensities. Indeed, increasing plasma fatty acid concentration during high-intensity endurance exercise via infusion of a lipid emulsion and heparin increases the rate of plasma fat oxidation [12]. However, the rate of fat oxidation is not fully restored under these conditions and the utilization of intramuscular triacylglycerol is still inhibited, and so it has not yet been clearly established whether delivery of fatty acids is a major factor limiting fat oxidation. The regulation of intramuscular triacylglycerol hydrolysis is being actively investigated at present. In addition, the transport of fatty acids across the muscle cell membrane and within the cell cytosol could be rate limiting. Recently, Smith et al. [13] suggested a key regulatory role for fatty acid translocase (FAT/CD36) in the entry of fatty acids into the cell and, more importantly, in delivery of fatty acids to acyl-CoA synthetase located near CPT1 on the outer mitochondrial membrane. However, this regulatory role of FAT/CD36 on fat oxidation has not yet been investigated at higher exercise intensities where rates of fat oxidation are known to decline, leaving no firm conclusions possible at this stage. Reactions distal to CPT1 which involve the limited intramitochondrial free coenzyme A pool (CoASH) such as CPT2 or various stages of the proximal β-oxidation pathway are also likely to be important regulators and require further investigation [14].

Despite the lack of knowledge of these other potential regulatory steps, there is increasing evidence to suggest that fat oxidation is indirectly regulated by flux through the pyruvate dehydrogenase complex (PDC) during exercise and that CPT1 is central to this regulation. For example, during exercise at 50% VO_2max, hyperglycemia (induced as a result of pre-exercise ingestion of glucose) increased glycolytic flux and reduced long-chain fatty acid ($[1-^{13}C]$palmitate) oxidation [15], whereas medium-chain $[1-^{13}C]$octanoate oxidation was unaffected. This suggests an inhibition of fat oxidation at the level of CPT1, as medium-chain fatty acids are oxidized independent of CPT1. Malonyl-CoA is a potent inhibitor of CPT1 activity in vitro and is a likely candidate as the intracellular regulator of the rate of long-chain fatty acid oxidation in human skeletal muscle, particularly as changes in muscle malonyl-CoA content have occurred with opposite changes in fat oxidation at rest [16]. However, despite a 122% increase in fat oxidation rates (due to depleted pre-exercise muscle glycogen content) during exercise at 65% VO_2peak, there were no differences in muscle malonyl-CoA content compared to control [17], suggesting that malonyl-CoA does not regulate CPT1 activity during exercise. Interestingly, a reduction in intracellular pH (from 7.1 to 6.8) in vitro reduces CPT1 activity by 34–40%, independent of any physiological change in malonyl-CoA concentration [18]. It is unlikely that this fall in pH would occur in vivo at the exercise intensity where the rate of fat oxidation routinely begins to decline, but it may suggest that changes in intracellular buffering could also play an important role in the regulation of the rate of fat oxidation. It has also been suggested that muscle contraction alters the sensitivity of CPT1 to malonyl-CoA and/or pH, but this would be difficult to test in vivo.

Role of Carnitine in the Regulation of Fat Oxidation

Carnitine is a major substrate for CPT1, and it has been hypothesized that the marked lowering of the muscle free carnitine pool during conditions of high PDC flux may limit CPT1 flux and thus the rate of fat oxidation [2, 19]. For example, during high-intensity endurance exercise, the rate of acetyl-CoA formation from PDC flux is in excess of its utilization by the tricarboxylic acid (TCA) cycle leading to its subsequent accumulation. Another role of carnitine in skeletal muscle is to buffer the excess acetyl groups formed, in a reaction catalyzed by carnitine acetyltransferase (CAT), to ensure that a viable pool of CoASH is maintained for the continuation of the PDC and TCA cycle reactions [19–22]. Indeed, following a few minutes of high-intensity exercise, the increase in acetylcarnitine formation is directly related to an increase in muscle acetyl-CoA [21]. Thus, van Loon et al. [2] demonstrated that a 35% decrease in the rate of fat oxidation that occurred at 72% VO_2max was paralleled by a 65% decline in skeletal muscle free carnitine content. Furthermore, the 2.5-fold decrease in the rate of fat oxidation during exercise at 65% VO_2max compared to control in the aforementioned study of Roepstorff et al. [17] coincided with a 50% reduction in free carnitine availability.

If we take all of these studies together, it is apparent that there is a dramatic decline in skeletal muscle free carnitine availability when it reaches 50% of the total carnitine pool at around 65% VO_2max (fig. 1). This exercise intensity coincides with that routinely reported at which fat oxidation begins to decline in healthy humans during cycling [3] and suggests that free carnitine availability becomes limiting to the rate of fat oxidation. However, it can also be seen from figure 1 that free carnitine availability declines at lower exercise intensities where rates of fat oxidation are still increasing. At first glance, this may suggest that free carnitine availability is not limiting to CPT1, but if we consider that β-oxidation will be increased several-fold at these low exercise intensities, then it could be predicted that the rate of acylcarnitine utilization by CPT2 will be increased, allowing increased CACT flux and intramitochondrial carnitine delivery to CPT1. When acetylation of the free carnitine pool reduces it availability to below 50% of the total pool, CACT also becomes limiting to the carnitine cycle flux, which would fit with the 1:1 stoichiometry of the CACT reaction and the fact that predicted intramitochondrial carnitine content at rest (equivalent of 0.5 mM intracellular water) is around double that of long-chain acylcarnitine (equivalent of 0.25 mM intracellular water) [23, 24]. Thus, free carnitine availability is limiting to CPT1 at any given exercise intensity and determined by flux through the CACT reaction, which in turn is limited by mitochondrial free carnitine availability above 65% VO_2max. With this in mind, increasing muscle total carnitine content could potentially increase the rate of fat oxidation during exercise, spare muscle glycogen, and increase exercise performance. Indeed, it is interesting to note that a significant positive association between total carnitine content and maximal activity of citrate synthase has been observed in skeletal muscle [25]. These observations may highlight an important link between mitochondrial oxidative capacity, intramitochondrial carnitine content, and the capacity for fat oxidation in skeletal muscle cells.

Effect of Increasing Skeletal Muscle Carnitine Availability on the Rate of Fat Oxidation

The majority of the pertinent studies in healthy humans to date have failed to increase skeletal muscle carnitine content via oral or intravenous L-carnitine administration [26]. For example, neither feeding L-carnitine daily for up 3 months [27], nor intravenously infusing L-carnitine for up to 5 h [28], had an effect on muscle total carnitine content, or indeed net uptake of carnitine across the leg [29]. Furthermore, feeding 2–5 g/day of L-carnitine for 1 week to 3 months prior to a bout of exercise, had no effect on perceived exertion, exercise performance, VO_2max, or markers of muscle substrate metabolism such as RER, VO_2, blood lactate, leg FFA turnover, and post exercise muscle glycogen content [26]. What was apparent from the earlier carnitine supplementation studies was that muscle carnitine content was either not measured or, if it was, not increased. This is likely explained by the finding that carnitine is transported into skeletal muscle against a considerable concentration gradient (>100-fold) which is saturated under normal conditions, and so it is unlikely that simply increasing plasma carnitine availability per se will increase muscle carnitine transport and storage [26]. However, insulin appears to stimulate skeletal muscle carnitine transport, and intravenously infusing L-carnitine in the presence of high circulating insulin (>50 mU/l) can increase muscle carnitine content by 15% [23, 28]. Furthermore, ingesting relatively large quantities of carbohydrate in a beverage (>80 g) can stimulate insulin release to a sufficient degree to increase whole-body carnitine retention when combined with 3 g of carnitine feeding and, if continued for up to 6 months (80 g carbohydrate + 1.36 g L-carnitine twice daily), can increase the muscle store by 20% compared to carbohydrate feeding alone [24].

Consistent with the hypothesis that free carnitine availability is limiting to CPT1 flux and fat oxidation, the increase in muscle total carnitine content in the study of Wall et al. [24] equated to an 80% increase in free carnitine availability during 30 min of exercise at 50% VO_2max compared to control and resulted in a 55% reduction in muscle glycogen utilization. Furthermore, this was accompanied by a 30% reduction in PDC activation status during exercise, suggesting that a carnitine-mediated increase in fat-derived acetyl-CoA inhibited PDC and muscle carbohydrate oxidation. Put another way, L-carnitine supplementation increased muscle free carnitine concentration during exercise at 50% VO_2max from 4.4 to 5.9 mM intracellular water, equating to an intramitochondrial concentration of 0.44 and 0.59 mM, which is below and above the K_m of CPT1 for carnitine, respectively [6]. The reduction in glycogen utilization could of course be due to an increase in plasma glucose disposal and utilization, which has been observed following carnitine feeding or intravenous infusion over periods which would not be expected to increase muscle total carnitine content [23, 30, 31], albeit under resting conditions. On the other hand, during 30 min of exercise at 80% VO_2max with increased muscle total carnitine content, the same apparent effects on fat oxidation were not observed [24]. In contrast, there was greater PDC activation (40%) and flux (16% greater acetylcarnitine), resulting in markedly reduced muscle lactate accumulation in the face of similar rates of glycogenolysis compared to control. This suggested that free carnitine availability was limiting to PDC flux during high-intensity exercise and that increasing muscle carnitine content resulted in a greater acetyl-CoA-buffering capacity and better matching of glycolytic to PDC flux. Furthermore, as free carnitine availability was not significantly greater than control during high-intensity exercise in the study of Wall et al. [24], and was below 50% of the total carnitine pool, it is likely that free carnitine delivery was still limiting to CPT1 and that, quantitatively, the CAT reaction (around 800 µmol/min per kg wet muscle over the first 3 min of exercise) 'stole' free carnitine from the CACT/CPT1 reaction (80 µmol/min per kg wet muscle at most).

Effect of Increasing Muscle Carnitine Content on Endurance Performance

The study by Wall et al. [24] also demonstrated a remarkable improvement in exercise performance in all participants (11% mean increase) during a 30-min cycle ergometer time trial in the carnitine-loaded state. This is consistent with animal studies reporting a delay in fatigue development by 25% during electrical stimulation in rat soleus muscle strips incubated in carnitine in vitro [32]. Whether these improvements in endurance performance are due to glycogen sparing as a result of a carnitine-mediated increase in fat oxidation or the reported effect of carnitine on glucose disposal requires further investigation, but due to the nature of the time trial, this seems unlikely. In fact, it is the reduced reliance on non-oxidative ATP production from carbohydrate oxidation (increase acetyl group buffering and reduced lactate accumulation) that is the more likely cause of the increased endurance performance observed [33]. Moreover, with the acetyl group buffering role of carnitine in mind, increasing muscle carnitine content may also allow a greater stockpiling of acetylcarnitine during a prior 'warm-up' exercise, which would then serve as a useful immediate supply of acetyl groups at the onset of a subsequent high-intensity performance task and again reduce the reliance on non-oxidative ATP production [34]. The beneficial effects of carnitine supplementation on glucose disposal may also aid with 'glycogen loading', which would likely influence performance during high-intensity endurance exercise [4]. Taken together, the long-held belief that carnitine supplementation can improve endurance performance via augmenting its role in fat oxidation should be revised to place more emphasis on the major role that carnitine plays in carbohydrate metabolism during exercise.

Acknowledgments

The studies described in this review from Dr. Francis B. Stephens and Dr. Benjamin Wall were conducted in Prof. Paul Greenhaff's Laboratory at the University of Nottingham, UK. The L-carnitine used in the studies was supplied by Lonza Ltd., Switzerland.

Disclosure Statement

The authors declare that no financial or other conflict of interest exists in relation to the content of the chapter.

References

1 Romijn JA, Coyle EF, Sidossis LS, et al: Relationship between fatty acid delivery and fatty acid oxidation during strenuous exercise. J Appl Physiol 1995;79:1939–1945.

2 van Loon LJ, Greenhaff PL, Constantin-Teodosiu D, et al: The effects of increasing exercise intensity on muscle fuel utilisation in humans. J Physiol 2001;536:295–304.

3 Achten J, Gleeson M, Jeukendrup AE: Determination of the exercise intensity that elicits maximal fat oxidation. Med Sci Sports Exerc 2002;34:92–97.

4 Bergstrom J, Hermansen L, Hultman E, Saltin B: Diet, muscle glycogen and physical performance. Acta Physiol Scand 1967;71:140–150.

5 Johnson RH, Walton JL, Krebs HA, Williamson RH: Metabolic fuels during and after severe exercise in athletes and non-athletes. Lancet 1969;2:452–455.

6 McGarry JD, Mills SE, Long CS, Foster DW: Observations on the affinity for carnitine, and malonyl-CoA sensitivity, of carnitine palmitoyltransferase I in animal and human tissues. Demonstration of the presence of malonyl-CoA in non-hepatic tissues of the rat. Biochem J 1983;214:21–28.

7 Fritz IB, Marquis NR: The role of acylcarnitine esters and carnitine palmityltransferase in the transport of fatty acyl groups across mitochondrial membranes. Proc Natl Acad Sci 1965;54:1226–1233.

8 McGarry JD, Brown NF: The mitochondrial carnitine palmitoyltransferase system. From concept to molecular analysis. Eur J Biochem 1997;244:1–14.

9 Cederblad G, Lindstedt S, Lundholm K: Concentration of carnitine in human muscle tissue. Clin Chim Acta 1974;53:311–321.

10 Fraser F, Zammit VA: Enrichment of carnitine palmitoyltransferases I and II in the contact sites of rat liver mitochondria. Biochem J 1998;329:225–229.

11 Idell-Wenger JA, Grotyohann LW, Neely JR: Coenzyme A and carnitine distribution in normal and ischemic hearts. J Biol Chem 1978;253:4310–4318.

12 Dyck DJ, Peters SJ, Wendling PS, et al: Regulation of muscle glycogen phosphorylase activity during intense aerobic cycling with elevated FFA. Am J Physiol 1996;270:E116–E125.

13 Smith BK, Bonen A, Holloway GP: A dual mechanism of action for skeletal muscle FAT/CD36 during exercise. Exerc Sport Sci Rev 2012;40:211–217.

14 Wall BT, Stephens FB, Marimuthu K, et al: Acute pantothenic acid and cysteine supplementation does not affect muscle coenzyme A content, fuel selection, or exercise performance in healthy humans. J Appl Physiol 2012;112:272–278.

15 Coyle EF, Jeukendrup AE, Wagenmakers AJ, Saris WH: Fatty acid oxidation is directly regulated by carbohydrate metabolism during exercise. Am J Physiol 1997;273:E268–E275.

16 Bavenholm PN, Pigon J, Saha AK, et al: Fatty acid oxidation and the regulation of malonyl-CoA in human muscle. Diabetes 2000;49:1078–1083.

17 Roepstorff C, Halberg N, Hillig T, et al: Malonyl-CoA and carnitine in regulation of fat oxidation in human skeletal muscle during exercise. Am J Physiol 2005;288:E133–E142.

18 Bezaire V, Heigenhauser GJ, Spriet LL: Regulation of CPT I activity in intermyofibrillar and subsarcolemmal mitochondria from human and rat skeletal muscle. Am J Physiol Endocrinol Metab 2004;286:E85–E91.

19 Harris RC, Foster CV, Hultman E: Acetylcarnitine formation during intense muscular contraction in humans. J Appl Physiol 1987;63:440–442.

20 Sahlin K: Muscle carnitine metabolism during incremental dynamic exercise in humans. Acta Physiol Scand 1990;138:259–262.

21 Constantin-Teodosiu D, Carlin JI, Cederblad G, et al: Acetyl group accumulation and pyruvate dehydrogenase activity in human muscle during incremental exercise. Acta Physiol Scand 1991;143:367–372.

22 Constantin-Teodosiu D, Cederblad G, Hultman E: PDC activity and acetyl group accumulation in skeletal muscle during prolonged exercise. J Appl Physiol 1992;73:2403–2407.

23 Stephens FB, Constantin-Teodosiu D, Laithwaite D, et al: An acute increase in skeletal muscle carnitine content alters fuel metabolism in resting human skeletal muscle. J Clin Endocrinol Metab 2006;91:5013–5018.

24 Wall BT, Stephens FB, Constantin-Teodosiu D, et al: Chronic oral ingestion of L-carnitine and carbohydrate increases muscle carnitine content and alters muscle fuel metabolism during exercise in humans. J Physiol 2011; 589:963–973.

25 Foster CV, Harris RC: Total carnitine content of the middle gluteal muscle of thoroughbred horses: normal values, variability and effect of acute exercise. Equine Vet J 1992;24:52–57.

26 Stephens FB, Constantin-Teodosiu D, Greenhaff PL: New insights concerning the role of carnitine in the regulation of fuel metabolism in skeletal muscle. J Physiol 2007;581:431–444.

27 Wächter S, Vogt M, Kreis R, et al: Long-term administration of L-carnitine to humans: effect on skeletal muscle carnitine content and physical performance. Clin Chim Acta 2002; 318:51–61.

28 Stephens FB, Constantin-Teodosiu D, Laithwaite D, et al: Insulin stimulates L-carnitine accumulation in human skeletal muscle. FASEB J 2006;20:377–379.

29 Soop M, Bjorkman O, Cederblad G, et al: Influence of carnitine supplementation on muscle substrate and carnitine metabolism during exercise. J Appl Physiol 1988;64: 2394–2399.

30 Galloway SD, Craig TP, Cleland SJ: Effects of oral L-carnitine supplementation on insulin sensitivity indices in response to glucose feeding in lean and overweight/obese males. Amino Acids 2011;41:507–515.

31 De Gaetano A, Mingrone G, Castagneto M, Calvani M: Carnitine increases glucose disposal in humans. J Am Coll Nutr 1999;18: 289–295.

32 Brass EP, Scarrow AM, Ruff LJ, et al: Carnitine delays rat skeletal muscle fatigue in vitro. J Appl Physiol 1993;75:1595–1600.

33 Timmons J, Poucher S, Constantin-Teodosiu D, et al: Metabolic responses from rest to steady state determine contractile function in ischemic skeletal muscle. Am J Physiol Endocrinol Metab 1997;273:E233–E238.

34 Campbell-O'Sullivan SP, Constantin-Teodosiu D, Peirce N, Greenhaff PL: Low intensity exercise in humans accelerates mitochondrial ATP production and pulmonary oxygen kinetics during subsequent more intense exercise. J Physiol 2002;538:931–939.

van Loon LJC, Meeusen R (eds): Limits of Human Endurance.
Nestlé Nutr Inst Workshop Ser, vol 76, pp 25–37, (DOI: 10.1159/000350225)
Nestec Ltd., Vevey/S. Karger AG., Basel, © 2013

Hydration during Intense Exercise Training

R.J. Maughan[a] · N.L. Meyer[b]

[a]Loughborough University, Loughborough, UK; [b]University of Colorado and
United States Olympic Committee, Colorado Springs, CO, USA

Abstract

Hydration status has profound effects on both physical and mental performance, and
sports performance is thus critically affected. Both overhydration and underhydration –
if sufficiently severe – will impair performance and pose a risk to health. Athletes may
begin exercise in a hypohydrated state as a result of incomplete recovery from water loss
induced in order to achieve a specific body mass target or due to incomplete recovery
from a previous competition or training session. Dehydration will also develop in endurance exercise where fluid intake does not match water loss. The focus has generally been
on training rather than on competition, but sweat loss and fluid replacement in training
may have important implications. Hypohydration may impair training quality and may
also increase stress levels. It is unclear whether this will have negative effects (reduced
training quality, impaired immunity) or whether it will promote a greater adaptive response. Hypohydration and the consequent hyperthermia, however, can enhance the
effectiveness of a heat acclimation program, resulting in improved endurance performance in warm and temperate environments. Drinking in training may be important in
enhancing tolerance of the gut when athletes plan to drink in competition. The distribution of water between body water compartments may also be important in the initiation
and promotion of cellular adaptations to the training stimulus.

Introduction

It is generally recognized that failure to maintain an adequate hydration status
will impair both physical and mental performance in a wide range of laboratory
tasks. There is some debate, though, as to the level of dehydration or

overhydration at which effects on performance become apparent, both in statistical terms and in terms of impairments that are meaningful for the athlete. This lack of consensus is hardly surprising, given the nature of the different exercise challenges used, the effects of varying environmental conditions, the different methods used to induce hypohydration, the varying characteristics of the subjects studied, and the individual variability in responses. There are also likely to be differences in the response depending on whether exercise begins with a pre-existing body water imbalance or whether dehydration develops as exercise progresses. Fluid replacement strategies during competition are also a matter of considerable controversy, with some advocating a planned strategy designed to limit the development of a water deficit or overload [1], while others insist that a simple reliance on thirst will ensure that the amount of fluid ingested is optimal [2, 3].

The focus of much of the available research has been on the consequences of a water deficit rather than water excess: the latter condition is uncommon and has generally been noted in very slow participants in marathon events or in other very prolonged activities. The focus of scientific interest has also been on the potential influence of hydration status on performance in sports competitions or on laboratory tasks intended to simulate the component physical and cognitive functions, but most athletes spend far more time in training than in competition. Elite rowers, for example, typically train for 4–6 h per day, but the event itself lasts a little over 6 min. Swimmers may train for 3–5 h per day for an event lasting less than 60 s. Hydration should therefore not be an issue in competition for these athletes unless they begin the event in a severely hypohydrated state, but substantial losses of water and electrolytes may be incurred in training. Even when the training duration is too short to cause major sweat losses, it is likely to be correspondingly more intense, and there will then be fluid redistribution between body water compartments: high-intensity exercise causes a substantial increase in the osmolality of the intracellular space of the active muscles and this will result in a corresponding decrease of the extracellular compartments, including the vascular space.

Notwithstanding the debate about the optimum hydration status and the most appropriate drinking strategy for athletes in competition, several considerations apply in relation to appropriate drinking behaviors in training. On the basis of the available information, it could be suggested that ensuring adequate hydration status would allow the athlete to maintain a high training load, in terms of intensity and volume, and thus maximize the training stimulus. Drinking in training would also allow the athlete to rehearse drinking strategies for competition, to practice the physical actions of drinking while engaging in the actions that characterize their sport, and to become accustomed to the sensation of exercising with fluids in the stomach. On the other hand, it could equally be suggested that training with a less than optimum hydration status would increase the physiological strain experienced by the athlete: this could have the effect of augmenting the training response, but also has the potential to increase the risk of illness or overtraining syndromes. With only limited evidence available, this analysis will attempt to evaluate which of these options might be more effective.

Water and Salt Balance in Training

The net fluid balance over a training session is determined by the rate of water loss and the amount of fluid ingested in training, and both loss and intake are influenced by many factors. Sweat losses are influenced by training intensity and duration, and by weather conditions, including temperature, humidity and wind speed, as well as by the practical considerations that dictate fluid availability. Drinks can be made available in essentially unlimited amounts in training for indoor sports and for some outdoor activities such as tennis or football training. Cyclists can carry some fluid with them without undue inconvenience or weight penalty. In running, however, it is unrealistic to carry significant amounts of fluid and few elite distance runners would ever expect to drink in training. Intake is also influenced by the preferences of the individual and the culture of the sport. The subjective response to the absence of fluid intake is likely to depend to a great extent on whether the athlete voluntarily chooses not to drink or whether this is imposed, either by the coach or by external circumstances.

Leiper et al. [4] used a deuterium tracer method to measure water turnover in a group of cyclists who covered an average of 50 (range 12–146) km/day in training at an average speed of 29 km/h in a cool (10°C) environment and in a sedentary group. Daily body mass remained essentially the same in both groups over the study period. Average median water turnover rate was faster ($p < 0.05$) in the cyclists (47 ml/kg per day, range 42–58) than the sedentary subjects (36 ml/kg per day, range 29–50; fig. 1). The average median daily urinary loss was similar in both groups, so the calculated non-renal daily water loss (comprising mostly sweat but also including respiratory, transcutaneous and fecal losses) was faster ($p < 0.05$) in the cyclists (19 ml/kg per day, range 13–35) than in the sedentary subjects (6 ml/kg per day, range 5–22), but there was no relationship between the average distance cycled daily and the water turnover rate. A report of fluid intake of elite Kenyan distance runners in training suggested that in spite of the absence of any fluid intake during the

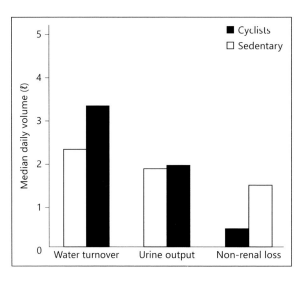

Fig. 1. Calculated average median daily water turnover rate, urine output and non-renal water loss for a group of cyclists in training and a sedentary group of subjects. Adapted from Leiper et al. [4].

one or two daily training sessions carried out, hydration status was well maintained over the 5-day study period [5]. Experience suggests that similar results would be obtained in other groups of athletes who choose not to drink in training: in spite of substantial fluid deficits incurred in each training session, there is not a progressive negative fluid balance over a period of days or weeks. This may imply that athletes make up for lost fluids after exercise and at meal times rather than during the actual training sessions, perhaps for reasons of convenience.

Even within a single group of athletes carrying out the same training session and with the same access to fluids, there can be a large difference in both sweating rate and drinking behavior. To illustrate the variability in response that is normally observed, some of the available data on sweat losses and fluid intake in elite male football players in training are summarized in table 1. All players in these studies were members of the first team squads at leading European clubs, and training was generally similar for each of the training sessions. Even though these players represent a rather homogeneous group, large individual differences in both sweating rates and drinking behaviors are apparent. Figure 2 shows the volume of fluid consumed in relation to the estimated sweat loss in elite football players in training: the response is highly variable, but, in this cohort of players, none drank so much that they gained weight. In a few players, the fluid intake was not sufficient to maintain body mass within 2% of the initial

Maughan · Meyer

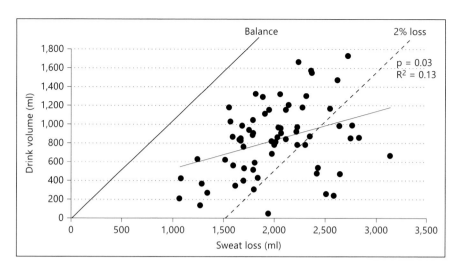

Fig. 2. The volume of fluid consumed and the sweat volume lost in training in several groups of football players. None of these players drank so much that they gained weight, but most drank sufficiently to limit body mass loss to less than 2% of the initial body mass. Data from various sources, including unpublished data. The line of balance would be where intake exactly matched loss so as to maintain the pre-training body mass.

Table 1. Sweat losses and fluid intake in elite professional football players

Temperature	Humidity, %	Players	Sweat loss, ml	Fluid intake, ml	Dehydration, %	Reference
32°C	20	26	2,193 (1,670–3,140)	972 (239–1,724)	1.59 (0.71–3.16)	[46]
27°C	55	24	2,033 (1,385–2,382)	971 (265–1,661)	1.37 (0.45–2.58)	[47]
28°C	56	20	2,221 (1,515–2,895)	1,401 (721–2,278)	1.15 (–0.24 to 2.30)	unpubl. data
25°C	60	24	1,827 (884–3,100)	834 (243–2,057)	1.22 (–0.24 to 2.60)	unpubl. data
5°C	81	16	1,690 (1,060–2,650)	423 (44–951)	1.62 (1.06–2.65)	[48]

All training sessions lasted about 90 min.

body mass. The sweat electrolyte concentration also varies greatly between individuals, and those who have high sweat rates, and high sweat sodium concentrations can lose substantial amounts of salt (sodium chloride) in training [6]. For some individuals, the losses in a single training session may far exceed the recommended daily salt intake.

Potassium is also lost in sweat. Sweat potassium concentration ranges from 5 to 10 mM [7], and this has been the basis for adding potassium to a sport beverage, typically at a concentration of about 5 mM. Sodium plays a critical role in restoring fluid balance after exercise; however, there is no evidence that the addition of potassium to drinks improves the restoration of fluid balance following dehydration, though restoration of potassium balance may be important for the maintenance of the intracellular water space [8, 9]. General guidelines for promoting recovery after exercise have focused on replacing sodium [1], with potassium mainly consumed through food (e.g. fruit, vegetables) later during the recovery process. As discussed later, though, cell volume may have important implications for both recovery from training and adaptation to the training stimulus.

Hydration Status and Stress Responses

Restriction of fluid intake during prolonged exercise results in increased core temperature, increased heart rate and increased perception of effort: there is also an increased plasma cortisol concentration during exercise when no fluid is ingested compared with trials where fluid is consumed [10]. These responses are likely to be amplified in warm environments. It might be argued that stress is an important element of the stimulus to adaptation, but because of the general suppression of immune function that usually accompanies elevated circulating cortisol levels, these observations raise concerns about a possible increased risk of infectious illness if hard training is performed consistently in a hypohydrated state. Some evidence to support this comes from a study on rats where intravenous endotoxin injection induced a febrile response in dehydrated rats but no such response was seen when the same endotoxin was injected into euhydrated rats [11]. There are data to show that even relatively mild (3% body mass loss) levels of dehydration can result in a decrease in the secretion rates of some of the salivary antimicrobial proteins that play an important role in mucosal immunity. Fortes et al. [12] reported decreased saliva secretion rates of lysozyme and α-amylase during prolonged exercise in the heat when no fluid was allowed, though the secretion rate of saliva secretory IgA remained unchanged. In the control trial, where sufficient fluid was consumed to replace sweat losses, there were no changes in secretion rates of any of the measured parameters.

Although a change in intestinal barrier function, with consequent increase in the risk of invading pathogens, might be postulated in the presence of hypohydration, Smetanka et al. [13] did not find any association between markers of gut barrier function and fractional body mass loss after a marathon race. Such cross-sectional studies, however, can provide only very limited information. A more recent review of gastrointestinal (GI) problems in athletes concluded that preventing dehydration might reduce the risk of GI complaints during intense exercise [14]. After the onset of exercise, splanchnic blood flow (SBF) decreases by about 20% at 10 min and by 80% after 1 h of exercise at 70% VO_2max [15]. This decrease in SBF is often cited as an important factor in the development of GI problems during exercise, especially in symptomatic athletes [16, 17]. Thus, the ingestion of fluid during exercise could have a protective effect on SBF and reduce the incidence of GI complaints during exercise. This may be important for those individuals who are especially prone to GI upset when training or competing.

Rehydration and Recovery between Training Bouts

The athlete's priorities for recovery after a training session will depend on several factors, but key among these is intensity and duration of the first session. This will determine the extent of substrate depletion and sweat losses, though the latter will also depend on environmental conditions and on the sweating characteristics of the individual. Also of critical importance is the time available for recovery before the next training session begins. Key considerations after endurance or team sports training are the replacement of carbohydrate stores in muscle and liver and restoration of water and salt balance [18]. Ensuring an appropriate nutrient, metabolic and hormonal environment to stimulate and support the adaptive response to the training stimulus is also a major objective for all athletes, as discussed in detail below.

The volume of water consumed after training should be sufficient to replace any net fluid deficit (the difference between water losses and water ingested) incurred during the training period. In addition, sufficient fluid should be ingested to allow for ongoing losses in sweat, expired breath and urine, and it is often recommended that the volume of fluid consumed in the immediate post-exercise period should be about 1.5 times the net fluid deficit [6]. Wong et al. [19] showed that a prescribed fluid intake was more effective than an ad libitum drinking schedule in restoring exercise capacity when applied during the 4-hour recovery period between two endurance exercise bouts. Even though the total fluid intake was the same on both trials, a greater volume was ingested in the early stages of recovery with the prescribed drinking schedule. The relative effects of the carbohydrate content of the drink and the fluid replacement could not, however, be separated with the study design used. Sufficient salt should be consumed to match sweat electrolyte losses and thus prevent a rapid diuresis: without restoration of salt balance, effective restoration of water balance cannot be achieved [20]. Water may be consumed in the form of a variety of beverages and foods, and the salt may come from food, if solid food is eaten, but in the absence of solid foods, drinks must provide sufficient electrolytes to replace net losses [21].

Training the Gut

The availability of ingested fluid is determined by the rates of gastric emptying and intestinal absorption. Either of these processes can limit the availability of ingested food and fluids. It has long been known that a high energy intake (i.e. regular intake of a high volume of food) is associated with a rapid mouth-to-caecum transit time [22]. There is some evidence that the rate of gastric emptying of liquids is not affected by a few days of ingestion of large volumes of liquids, but subjective reports of gastric comfort show that tolerance develops rapidly [Leiper and Maughan, unpubl. data]. In addition, limited evidence shows that gastric emptying rates may be increased with endurance training [23].

The absorptive capacity of the gut is capable of rapid adaptation to periods of feeding and fasting, and is highly responsive to changes in the composition of the diet. The maximum rates of carbohydrate absorption that can be achieved may be enhanced by a short period of adaptation to a high carbohydrate diet [24]. In a study of highly trained athletes, a group who consumed glucose during each of their workouts over a 4-week training block increased their ability to oxidize this carbohydrate, while muscle oxidation of carbohydrate consumed during exercise remained constant in a matched group who did the same training with ingestion of water [25]. The design of this study could not distinguish whether the adaptation was achieved by a higher intake of carbohydrate or in response to the specific intake of the carbohydrate during exercise. An increased capacity to absorb carbohydrate may be important from a hydration perspective as carbohydrate uptake in the intestine can drive the movement of water from the intestinal lumen into the circulation [26].

These data suggest that athletes in endurance events may benefit from specific efforts to increase tolerance to large volumes of carbohydrate-containing fluid in the gut and to enhance the rate at which ingested water and substrate can be absorbed into the circulation. Further, higher amounts of carbohydrate may be tolerated during prolonged exercise if attention is given to the type of carbohydrate (e.g. glucose and fructose) [27].

Finally, the temperature of the drinks that are consumed during exercise is also important, especially when training in the heat. A recent meta-analysis

Maughan · Meyer

shows that beverages with a temperature <22°C significantly increase palatability of the fluid, with consequent effects on the volume of fluid consumed and on hydration status during exercise [28].

Adaptation to Dehydration and Coping Strategies

Some athletes and coaches deliberately restrict fluid intake in training in the belief that the body will adapt to a lack of fluid and will therefore cope better with dehydration in competition. Deliberate restriction of fluid intake has long been a common practice in sport [29] and added to this the use of purgatives, laxatives and 'sweating liquors' was also common among early athletes to promote weight loss [30]. Practices in many sports have changed substantially, but particularly in the weight category or weight-sensitive sports, where acute dehydration is a normal part of pre-competition preparation for the majority of competitors, chronic hypohydration is not uncommon [31]. Even when fluids are provided, it is common for athletes in weight category sports to drink little or nothing during training, perhaps in the belief that they will adapt to the dehydrated state [32]. There is no evidence that the body adapts to dehydration, although those who frequently restrict fluid intake may learn to complain less about the symptoms that accompany it. It is perhaps also likely that those who are resistant to the effects of dehydration are those who persist in participation in weight category sports. Those who cannot tolerate the weight-making process are likely to discontinue participation in the sport.

Dehydration during training may, however, enhance the effectiveness of a short-term heat acclimation program in both untrained individuals and in highly trained athletes [33]. This seems to be a consequence of the greater elevation of core temperature that occurs when exercising in the heat in a hypohydrated state and the consequently greater cardiovascular adaptations that ensue, including the extent of the increase in vascular volume [34, 35]. Emerging evidence suggests that the adaptations that occur in response to even a short period of heat acclimation may promote enhanced endurance performance in a temperate environment [36].

Hydration and Adaptation to Training

The aim of training is, or should be, to enhance performance in competition. To achieve this, the training stimulus must induce a selective expression of the genetic potential of the individual. There must be a selective stimulation of protein synthesis and breakdown so that the tissue content of proteins that convey a performance advantage is increased. For the strength athlete, this may mean an increase in the muscle content of the contractile proteins, actin and myosin: for the marathon runner, an increase in muscle mass would be a disadvantage, so the aim is to increase the muscle content of mitochondrial protein and this an increase in oxidative capacity. These are examples only, and a complex pattern of tissue remodeling takes place in response to training. There has been considerable focus on the nutritional strategies that can promote these changes, especially on the provision of protein [37].

The potential role of hydration status in modulating the response to training has been largely ignored, but hard training can not only induce substantial fluid deficits, it can also result in large movements of fluid between body water compartments. Changes in the water content of cells can have a large effect on all aspects of cell function. In short-term high-intensity exercise, there is a large increase in intracellular osmolality in the active muscles as glycogen is broken down to lower molecular weight intermediates, and other complex molecules are degraded. In spite of the existence of compensatory mechanisms that attempt to prevent changes in cell volume, the high intracellular osmotic pressure causes water to move from the extracellular space into the active muscles, resulting in cell swelling. Raja et al. [38] showed a 13% increase in the intracellular water content of forearm muscle during intensive forearm wrist flexion exercise. In high-intensity running or cycling exercise, the increase in the water content of the active muscles is likely to be even higher because of the greater accumulation of metabolic intermediates, and intense cycling exercise is accompanied by a decrease in plasma volume of 20–25% or even more [39].

Major disturbances of cell volume have profound effects on cellular metabolism [40]. Cell swelling will favor anabolic reactions, including protein synthesis and glycogen synthesis, while cell shrinkage will encourage these reactions to proceed in the opposite direction [41]. The expansion of cell volume after intense exercise may therefore play an important role in the initiation and regulation of the changes in protein synthesis that must occur in order to produce the functional changes that accompany training. It may be worth noting that the ratio of intracellular to extracellular water also falls with age [42], and this may be relevant to the generally observed reduction in the capacity of the older individual to respond to a training stimulus. At present, however, our understanding of the influence of cell volume changes on regulatory pathways does not allow practical recommendations to be made [43]. Finally, it is important to understand that water intake per se does not equate to cell swelling, as these processes are much more complex [40].

In summary, training in the hydrated state and/or resuming euhydration as soon as possible after exercise seem to be more appropriate strategies to support training adaptation than training in a hypohydrated state, although insufficient data are available to permit firm conclusions.

Practical Implications

Optimizing hydration practices in athletes should be initiated via education and individual hydration status and sweat rate assessments. Sweat rates can be assessed fairly well using body mass changes, although some limitations exist. Respiratory water loss, substrate oxidation and mass loss, as well as changes in body water due to fluid intake and urinary or fecal loss all contribute to errors when estimating sweat rate from changes in body mass [44]. However, by measuring fluid intake, selecting critical exercise sessions, and repeating these measurements in various environments, estimates of sweat rates can be determined fairly well from body mass changes. It is worth remembering that most investigations into the effects of sweat loss on exercise performance have used body mass loss as the measure of sweat loss, so it is not inappropriate to advise athletes on the basis of body mass loss.

Athletes often begin training in the dehydrated state. Assessing urine osmolality or specific gravity can be helpful in establishing a baseline and initiate good drinking behavior in athletes. However, urinary measures are likely to be unreliable after exercise as changes lag behind the changes occurring in the plasma [46]. Sport nutrition practitioners may use these strategies to establish hydration status and sweat rates, and improve athletes' knowledge and skills pertaining to the individualization of hydration strategies. Too often, however, these strategies can create an athlete dependency on such services.

While it may be useful to determine individual sweat rates, it appears equally important to teach the athlete to increase tolerance to greater fluid volumes and higher carbohydrate intakes, especially for prolonged exercise and exercise in the heat. If changes in fluid consumption should impact performance at competitions, practice to drink should be integrated into high-intensity training sessions. It is expected that the GI system adapts with repeated exposures to drinking in training.

Disclosure Statement

R.J.M. is Chair of the Science Advisory Board of the European Hydration Institute.

References

1 Sawka MN, Burke LM, Eichner ER, et al: Exercise and fluid replacement. Med Sci Sports Exerc 2007;39:377–390.

2 Noakes TD: Hydration in the marathon: using thirst to gauge safe fluid replacement. Sports Med 2007;37:463–466.

3 Noakes TD: Waterlogged. Champaign, Human Kinetics, 2012.

4 Leiper JB, Pitsiladis Y, Maughan RJ: Comparison of water turnover rates in men undertaking prolonged cycling exercise and in sedentary men. Int J Sports Med 2001;22:181–185.

5 Fudge B, Easton C, Kingsmore D, et al: Elite Kenyan endurance runners are hydrated day-to-day with ad libitum fluid intake. Med Sci Sports Exerc 2008;40:1171–1179.

6 Shirreffs SM, Sawka MN: Fluid and electrolyte needs for training, competition, and recovery. J Sports Sci 2011;29:S39–S46.

7 Maughan RJ, Shirreffs SM: Recovery from prolonged exercise: restoration of water and electrolyte balance. J Sport Sci 1997;15:297–303.

8 Nielsen B, Sjøgaard G, Ugelvig J, et al: Fluid balance in exercise dehydration and rehydration with different glucose-electrolyte drinks. Eur J Appl Physiol 1986;55:318–325.

9 Maughan RJ, Owen JH, Shirreffs SM, Leiper JB: Post-exercise rehydration in man: effects of electrolyte addition to ingested fluids. Eur J Appl Physiol Occup Physiol 1994;69:209–215.

10 Bishop NC, Scanlon GA, Walsh NP, et al: No effect of fluid intake on neutrophil responses to prolonged cycling. J Sports Sci 2004;22:1091–1098.

11 Morimoto A, Murakami N, Ono T, Watanabe T: Dehydration enhances endotoxin fever by increased production of endogenous pyrogen. Am J Physiol 1986;251:R41–R47.

12 Fortes MB, Diment BC, Di Felice U, Walsh NP: Dehydration decreases saliva antimicrobial proteins important for mucosal immunity. Appl Physiol Nutr Metab 2012;37:1–10.

13 Smetanka RD, Lambert GP, Murray R, et al: Intestinal permeability in runners in the 1996 Chicago Marathon. Int J Sport Nutr 1999;9:426–433.

14 ter Steege RWF, Kolkman JJ: Review article: the pathophysiology and management of gastrointestinal symptoms during physical exercise, and the role of splanchnic blood flow. Aliment Pharmacol Ther 2012;35:516–528.

15 Rehrer NJ, Smets A, Reynaert H, et al: Effect of exercise on portal vein blood flow in man. Med Sci Sports Exerc 2001;33:1533–1537.

16 ter Steege RWT, Geelkerken RH, Huisman AB, Kolkman JJ: Abdominal symptoms during physical exercise and the role of gastrointestinal ischaemia: a study in 12 symptomatic athletes. Br J Sports Med 2012;46:931–935.

17 van Nieuwenhoven MA, Brouns F, Brummer RJ: Gastrointestinal profile of symptomatic athletes at rest and during physical exercise. Eur J Appl Physiol 2004;91:429–434.

18 Spaccarotella KJ, Andzel WD: Building a beverage for recovery from endurance activity: a review. J Strength Cond Res 2011;25:3198–3204.

19 Wong SH, Williams C, Simpson M, et al: Influence of fluid intake pattern on short-term recovery from prolonged, submaximal running and subsequent exercise capacity. J Sports Sci 1998;16:143–152.

20 Shirreffs, SM, Taylor AJ, Leiper JB, Maughan RJ: Post-exercise rehydration in man: effects of volume consumed and drink sodium content. Med Sci Sports Exerc 1996;28:1260–1271.

21 Maughan RJ, Leiper JB, Shirreffs SM: Restoration of fluid balance after exercise-induced dehydration: effects of food and fluid intake. Eur J Appl Physiol 1996;73:317–325.

22 Harris A, Lindeman AK, Martin BJ: Rapid orocecal transit in chronically active persons with high-energy intake. J Appl Physiol 1991;70:1550–1553.

23 Gisolfi CV: Is the GI system built for exercise? News Physiol Sci 2000;15:114–119.

24 Jeukendrup AE, McLaughlin J: Carbohydrate ingestion during exercise: Effects on performance, training adaptations and trainability of the gut; in Maughan RJ, Burke LM (eds): Sports Nutrition: More Than Just Calories – Triggers for Adaptation. Nestlé Nutr Inst Workshop Ser. Nestec, Vevey/Karger, Basel, 2011, vol 69, pp 1–17.

25 Cox GR, Clark SA, Cox AJ, et al: Daily training with high carbohydrate availability increases exogenous carbohydrate oxidation during endurance cycling. J Appl Physiol 2010;109:126–134.

26 Schedl HP, Maughan RJ, Gisolfi CV: Intestinal absorption during rest and exercise: implications for formulating oral rehydration beverages. Med Sci Sports Ex 1994;26:267–280.

27 Jeukendrup AE: Nutrition for endurance sports: marathon, triathlon, and road cycling. J Sports Sci 2011;29(suppl 1):S91–S99.

28 Burdon CA, Johnson NA, Chapman PG, O'Connor HT: Influence of beverage temperature on palatability and fluid ingestion during endurance exercise: a systematic review. Int J Sport Nutr Exerc Metab 2012;22:199–211.

29 Downer AR: Running Recollections and How to Train. London, Gale and Polden, 1902.

30 Thom W: Pedestrianism. Aberdeen, Chalmers, 1813.

31 Wilson G, Chester N, Eubank M: An alternative dietary strategy to make weight while improving mood, decreasing body fat, and not dehydrating: a case study of a professional jockey. Int J Sport Nutr Exerc Metab 2012; 22:225–231.

32 Rivera-Brown AM, De Felix-Davila RA: Hydration status in adolescent judo athletes before and after training in the heat. Int J Sport Physiol Perf 2012;7:39–46.

33 Garrett AT, Creasy R, Rehrer NJ: Effectiveness of short-term heat acclimation for highly trained athletes. Eur J Appl Physiol 2012;112: 1827–1837.

34 Fan J-L, Cotter JD, Lucas RAI, et al: Human cardiorespiratory and cerebrovascular function during severe passive hyperthermia: effects of mild hypohydration. J Appl Physiol 2008;105:433–445.

35 Ikegawa S, Kamijo J, Okazaki K, et al: Effects of hypohydration on thermoregulation during exercise before and after 5-day aerobic training in a warm environment in young men. J Appl Physiol 2011;110:972–980.

36 Lorenzo S, Halliwill JR, Sawka MN, Minson CT: Heat acclimation improves exercise performance. J Appl Physiol 2010;109:1140–1147.

37 van Loon LJC, Gibala M: Dietary protein to support muscle hypertrophy; in Maughan RJ, Burke LM (eds): Sports Nutrition: More Than Just Calories – Triggers for Adaptation. Nestlé Nutr Inst Workshop Ser. Nestec, Vevey/Karger, Basel, 2011, vol 69, pp 79–96.

38 Raja MK, Raymer MH, Moran GR, et al: Changes in tissue water content measured with multiple-frequency bioimpedance and metabolism measured with P-31-MRS during progressive forearm exercise. J Appl Physiol 2006;101:1070–1075.

39 Nose H, Takamata A, Mack GW, et al: Water and electrolyte balance in the vascular space during graded-exercise in humans. J Appl Physiol 1991;70:2757–2762.

40 Lang F: Effect of cell hydration on metabolism; in Maughan RJ, Burke LM (eds): Sports Nutrition: More Than Just Calories – Triggers for Adaptation. Nestlé Nutr Inst Workshop Ser. Nestec, Vevey/Karger, Basel, 2011, vol 69, pp 115–130.

41 Lang F, Busch GL, Ritter M, et al: Functional significance of cell volume regulatory mechanisms. Physiol Rev 1998;78:247–306.

42 Adolph EF: Origins of Physiological Regulations. New York, Academic Press, 1968.

43 Maughan RJ, Burke LM: Practical nutritional recommendations for the athlete; in Maughan RJ, Burke LM (eds): Sports Nutrition: More Than Just Calories – Triggers for Adaptation. Nestlé Nutr Inst Workshop Ser. Nestec, Vevey/Karger, Basel, 2011, vol 69, pp 131–149.

44 Maughan RJ, Shirreffs SM, Leiper JB: Errors in the estimation of hydration status from changes in body mass. J Sports Sci 2007;25: 797–804.

45 Shirreffs SM, Taylor AJ, Leiper JB, Maughan RJ: Post-exercise rehydration in man: effects of volume consumed and sodium content of ingested fluids. Med Sci Sports Exerc 1996; 28:1260–1271.

46 Shirreffs SM, Aragon-Vargas LF, Chamorro M, et al: The sweating response of elite professional soccer players to training in the heat. Int J Sports Med 2005;26:90–95.

47 Shirreffs SM, Sawka MN, Stone M: Water and electrolyte needs for football training and match-play. J Sports Sci 2006;24:699–707.

48 Maughan RJ, Shirreffs SM, Merson SJ, Horswill CA: Fluid and electrolyte balance in elite male football (soccer) players training in a cool environment. J Sports Sci 2005;23: 73–79.

van Loon LJC, Meeusen R (eds): Limits of Human Endurance.
Nestlé Nutr Inst Workshop Ser, vol 76, pp 39–50, (DOI: 10.1159/000350254)
Nestec Ltd., Vevey/S. Karger AG., Basel, © 2013

Intense Exercise Training and Immune Function

Michael Gleeson · Clyde Williams

School of Sport, Exercise and Health Sciences, Loughborough University, Loughborough, UK

Abstract

Regular moderate exercise reduces the risk of infection compared with a sedentary life-style, but very prolonged bouts of exercise and periods of intensified training are associated with increased infection risk. In athletes, a common observation is that symptoms of respiratory infection cluster around competitions, and even minor illnesses such as colds can impair exercise performance. There are several behavioral, nutritional and training strategies that can be adopted to limit exercise-induced immunodepression and minimize the risk of infection. Athletes and support staff can avoid transmitting infections by avoiding close contact with those showing symptoms of infection, by practicing good hand, oral and food hygiene and by avoiding sharing drinks bottles and cutlery. Medical staff should consider appropriate immunization for their athletes particularly when travelling to international competitions. The impact of intensive training stress on immune function can be minimized by getting adequate sleep, minimizing psychological stress, avoiding periods of dietary energy restriction, consuming a well-balanced diet that meets energy and protein needs, avoiding deficiencies of micronutrients (particularly iron, zinc, and vitamins A, D, E, B_6 and B_{12}), ingesting carbohydrate during prolonged training sessions, and consuming – on a daily basis – plant polyphenol containing supplements or foodstuffs and *Lactobacillus* probiotics.

Introduction

A person's level of physical activity influences his/her risk of infection, most likely by affecting immune function. Regular moderate exercise reduces the risk of infection compared with a sedentary lifestyle [1, 2], but very prolonged bouts of exercise and periods of intensified training are associated with increased infection risk. Acute bouts of exercise cause a temporary depression of various aspects of immune function that will usually last for up to 24 h after exercise, depending on the intensity and duration of the exercise bout [3]. Several studies indicate that the incidence of symptoms of upper respiratory tract illness (URTI) is increased in the days after prolonged strenuous endurance events [4, 5], and it has been generally assumed that this reflects the temporary depression of immune function induced by prolonged exercise. More recently, it has been proposed that at least some of the symptoms of URTI in athletes are attributable to upper airway inflammation rather than to infectious episodes [6]. Periods of intensified training lasting a week or more have been shown to depress immune function [7], and although elite athletes are not clinically immune deficient, it is possible that the combined effects of small changes in several immune factors may compromise resistance to common minor illnesses, particularly during periods of prolonged heavy training and at times of major competitions.

Causes of Illness in Athletes

The most common illnesses in athletes (and in the general population) are viral infections of the upper respiratory tract (i.e. the common cold) which are more common in the winter months, and adults typically experience 2–4 URTI episodes per year. Athletes can also develop similar symptoms (e.g. sore throat) due to allergy or inflammation caused by inhalation of cold, dry or polluted air [7]. In themselves, these symptoms are generally trivial, but no matter whether the cause is infectious or allergic inflammation, they can cause an athlete to interrupt training, underperform or even miss an important competition. A recent survey of hundreds of elite GB athletes in 30 different Olympic sports reported that among the reasons for athletes having to miss training sessions in 33% of cases, it was because of infection (most commonly URTI). Recent analysis of the 126 reported illnesses in athletes competing in the 2011 World Athletics Championships in Daegu, South Korea, revealed that 40% of illnesses affected the upper respiratory tract with confirmed infection in about 20% of cases [8]. Other main causes of sickness were associated with exercise-induced dehydration (12% of cases) and gastroenteritis/diarrhea (10% of cases).

Prolonged bouts of strenuous exercise have been shown to result in transient depression of white blood cell functions, and it is suggested that such changes create an 'open window' of decreased host protection, during which viruses and bacteria can gain a foothold, increasing the risk of developing an infection [3]. Other factors such as psychological stress, lack of sleep and malnutrition can also depress immunity [9] and lead to increased risk of infection (fig. 1). There are also some situations in which an athlete's exposure to infectious agents may be increased,

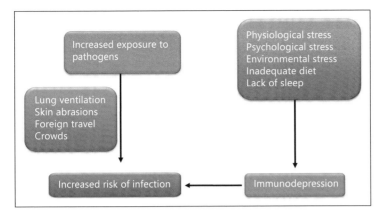

Fig. 1. Causes of increased infection risk in athletes.

which is the other important determinant of infection risk. During exercise, exposure to airborne bacteria and viruses increases because of the higher rate and depth of breathing. An increase in gut permeability may also allow entry of gut bacterial endotoxins into the circulation, particularly during prolonged exercise in the heat. In contact sports, skin abrasions may occur increasing the risk of transdermal infections. In some sports, the competitors may be in close proximity to large crowds. Air travel to foreign countries may be involved. Hence, the cause of the increased incidence of infection in athletes is most likely multifactorial (fig. 1). A variety of stressors (physical, psychological, environmental, and nutritional) may suppress immune function, and these effects, together with increased exposure to potentially disease-causing pathogens, can make the athlete more susceptible to infection. There appears to be no influence of the sex of an athlete on susceptibility to URTI [10] but some athletes are more illness-prone than others.

Intensive Training Effects on Immune Function

Prolonged bouts of strenuous exercise have a temporary negative impact on immune function. Post-exercise immune function depression is most pronounced when the exercise is continuous, prolonged (>1.5 h), of moderate to high intensity (55–75% of aerobic capacity), and performed without food intake [11]. Both aspects of innate immunity (e.g. neutrophil chemotaxis, phagocytosis, degranulation and oxidative burst activity, monocyte toll-like receptor expression and natural killer cell cytoxic activity) and acquired immunity (e.g. antigen presentation by monocytes/macrophages, T lymphocyte cytokine production and proliferation, immunoglobulin production by B lymphocytes) are depressed by prolonged exercise. The salivary secretory immunoglobulin A (SIgA) response to acute exercise is variable, though very prolonged bouts of exercise are commonly reported to result in decreased SIgA secretion [12]. The causes of immune depression after prolonged exercise are thought to be related to increases in circulating stress hormones (e.g. adrenaline and cortisol), alterations in the pro-/anti-inflammatory cytokine balance and increased oxidative stress.

Markers of immune function in athletes in the true resting state (i.e. at least 24 h after the last exercise bout) are generally not very different from their sedentary counterparts, except when athletes are engaged in periods of intensified training. In this situation, immune function might not fully recover from successive training sessions and some functions can become chronically depressed [7]. Both T and B lymphocyte functions appear to be sensitive to increases in training load in well-trained athletes undertaking a period of intensified training, with decreases in circulating numbers of type 1 T cells, inhibition of type 1 T cell cytokine production, reduced T cell proliferative responses and falls in stimulated B cell immunoglobulin synthesis and SIgA reported. However, to date, the only immune variable that has been consistently associated with increased infection incidence is SIgA. Low concentrations of SIgA in athletes or substantial transient falls in SIgA are associated with increased risk of URTI [13]. In contrast, increases in SIgA can occur after a period of regular moderate exercise training in previously sedentary individuals and could, at least in part, contribute to the apparent reduced susceptibility to URTI associated with regular moderate exercise compared with a sedentary lifestyle [3].

The prevention of infection is vitally important research area both in terms of the health of the population at large and particularly for athletes undertaking prolonged periods of heavy training. In terms of negative impact on training, repeated periods of infection are akin to recurrent physical injuries which can be catastrophic when they occur as athletes approach major competitions. Therefore, the study by Neville et al. [13] is particularly encouraging because it showed on retrospective analyses of the salivary samples of 38 Americas Cup athletes taken over 50 weeks that when their relative IgA values fell by 40% or more they were likely to experience infections within a week or two. With the impending availability of rapid 'in the field' salivary analysis using hand-held devices, these measurements may offer a way of informing coaches when athletes are most vulnerable to infection and so infection problems associated with increased training loads might be avoided.

The available, albeit limited, evidence does not support the contention that athletes training and competing in cold conditions experience a greater reduction in immune function compared with thermoneutral conditions [3]. The inhalation of cold dry air can reduce upper airway ciliary movement and decrease mucous flow, but it remains unknown if athletes who regularly train and compete in cold conditions report more frequent, severe or longer-lasting infections. Other environmental extremes (e.g. heat and altitude) or dehydration do not seem to have a marked impact on immune responses to exercise [3].

Infections can occur following exposure to new pathogens, but can also be caused by reactivation of a latent virus. For example, it has been shown that symptoms of URTI in swimmers were positively associated with previous infection with Epstein-Barr virus and partially with viral shedding [14]. Prior infection with cytomegalovirus may also have a similar effect. Both these viruses produce a homologue of interleukin-10, a potent anti-inflammatory cytokine which impairs the body's ability to mount an effective immune response to pathogenic challenges.

Recently, in a collaboration with researchers from the Anthony Nolan Research Institute (London), we have compared the levels of T cell receptor excision circles (TREC), a marker of recent thymic emigrants, as well as the levels of circulating lymphocyte subsets in a group of elite triathletes and in age-matched controls [15]. This analysis revealed that the concentration of TREC molecules in the athletes was significantly lower than in age-matched controls, and the athletes also had far fewer naïve T cells. Thymus function declines with age, and while the output of both TREC and naïve T cells is relatively constant in the first 3 decades after birth, there is a significant decline observable from the late 20s to 30 years of age. Values as low as those seen in the athletes are not normally observed in normal individuals until they reach at least 60 years of age. Athletes prolonging their careers into their 30s (or beyond) may run the risk of passing from an exercise-induced thymic deficiency to an age-dependent one, creating a permanent distortion, in effect a premature ageing, in their peripheral T cell repertoire that leaves them at reduced capacity to respond to new infectious challenges. Such changes could also increase autoimmunity, as is seen in ageing. The extent to which these effects on the immune system persist on cessation of exercise training is not known, and is clearly of importance to establish if the long-term health of athletes is to be protected.

Practical Guidelines to Maintain Immune Health and Limit the Risk of Infection

It is generally agreed that prevention is always preferable to treatment, and although there is no single method that completely eliminates the risk of contracting an infection, there are several effective behavioral, nutritional and training strategies that can reduce the extent of exercise-induced immunodepression and lower the risk of infection [9], and these are summarized in figure 2.

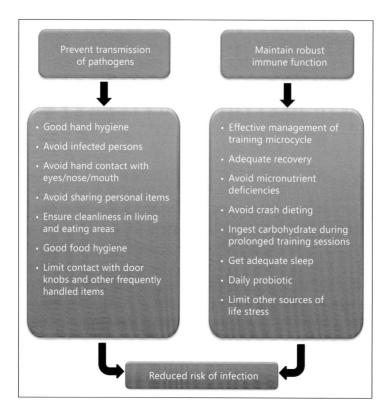

Fig. 2. Strategies to limit the risk of infection in athletes.

Some practical guidelines to limit transmission of infections among athletes are shown in table 1. The most important of these are good hand hygiene and avoiding contact with persons that are infected. Hand washing (with the correct technique to ensure all parts of hands are cleaned effectively) with soap and water is effective against most pathogens but does not provide continuous protection. Hand gels containing >60% alcohol disinfect effectively but the protection they provide does not last long (only a few minutes), so they need to be applied frequently and this can cause skin drying and irritation. Other sanitization methods include the use of non-alcohol based antimicrobial hand foams (e.g. Byotrol products which contain a mixture of cationic biocides and hydrophobic polymers) that are claimed to disinfect hands for up to 6 h. However, individuals need to be aware that these products are removed by hand washing and excessive sweating and so really need to be reapplied every few hours.

The other things that athletes can do to limit their risk of infection are to adhere to some practical guidelines to maintain robust immunity and limit the impact of training stress. These guidelines (table 2) relate mostly to nutritional,

Table 1. Guidelines to limit transmission of infections among athletes

– Individuals should be updated on all vaccines needed at home and for foreign travel. Influenza vaccines take 5–7 weeks to take effect; intramuscular vaccines may have a few small side effects, so it is advisable to vaccinate out of season. Don't vaccinate just before competitions or if symptoms of illness are present.
– Minimize contact with infected people, young children, animals and contagious objects.
– Keep at distance to people who are coughing, sneezing or have a 'runny nose', and when appropriate wear (or ask them to wear) a disposable mask.
– Quickly isolate an individual with infection symptoms from others.
– Protect airways from being directly exposed to very cold (<–10°C) and dry air during strenuous exercise by using a facial mask.
– Wash hands regularly, before meals, and after direct contact with potentially contagious people, animals, blood, secretions, public places and bathrooms.
– Use disposable paper towels and limit hand to mouth/nose contact when suffering from respiratory or gastrointestinal infection symptoms (putting hands to eyes and nose is a major route of viral self-inoculation).
– Carry alcohol-based hand-washing gel with you.
– Do not share drinking bottles, cups, cutlery, towels etc. with other people.
– While competing or training abroad, choose cold beverages from sealed bottles, avoid raw vegetables and undercooked meat. Wash and peel fruit before eating.

training and recovery strategies and are based on the findings of numerous research studies; only some of the more important ones are cited as examples in table 2. The most effective nutritional strategies to maintain robust immune function during intensive training are to avoid deficiencies of essential micronutrients, ingest carbohydrate during exercise and ingest *Lactobacillus* probiotics on a daily basis. While not all probiotics have been shown to help maintain healthy levels of salivary IgA, prolonged ingestion of some *Lactobacillus* strains has provided encouraging results [16]. Therefore, athletes should be advised on how best to fortify their diets with the appropriate type of probiotic.

In addition to obeying the rules of good personal hygiene, the composition of the diet and timing of food intake may also help provide protection against infections. Recognizing that after heavy training and competition immune function is compromised and that carbohydrate, protein and fluid ingestion helps restore function [17–19], it is even more important that athletes are encouraged to develop feeding strategies that focus on the post-exercise period as part of their overall nutritional plans.

When cold symptoms begin, there is some evidence that taking zinc lozenges at this time (>75 mg zinc/day; high ionic zinc content) can reduce the number of days that illness symptoms last for. Ensuring that the individual has adequate

Table 2. Guidelines to help maintain robust immunity and limit training stress

– Ensure adequate dietary energy, protein and essential micronutrient intake. It has only recently been recognized that vitamin D plays an important role in upregulating immunity [22], and this is a concern as vitamin D insufficiency is common in athletes [20], especially if exposure to natural sunlight is limited (e.g. when training in the winter months or when training mostly indoors). An increasing number of studies in athletes and the general population indicate that sufficient vitamin D status optimizes immune function and defends against respiratory infections. Thus, athletes who have deficient or insufficient vitamin D status are likely to benefit from supplementation and monitoring of circulating 25-hydroxy vitamin D concentration in athletes at risk of insufficiency is warranted.

– Avoid crash dieting and rapid weight loss. Care should be taken to ensure adequate protein (and micronutrient) intakes during periods of intentional weight loss, and it should be recognized that athletes undergoing weight reduction are likely to be more prone to infection. In general, a broad-range multivitamin/mineral supplement is the best choice to support a restricted food intake, and this may also be suitable for the travelling athlete in situations where food choices and quality may be limited.

– Ensure adequate carbohydrate intake before and during strenuous prolonged exercise in order to limit the extent and severity of exercise-induced immunodepression. Carbohydrate ingestion during exercise limits metabolic stress by helping to maintain the blood glucose concentration. The use of a high-carbohydrate diet and carbohydrate ingestion (about 30–60 g/h) during prolonged workouts lowers circulating stress hormone (e.g. adrenaline and cortisol) and anti-inflammatory cytokine (e.g. interleukins 6 and 10) responses to exercise and delays the appearance of symptoms of overreaching during intensive training periods [23]. This reduces the impact of prolonged exercise on several, but not all, aspects of immune function although evidence is currently lacking to demonstrate that this translates to a reduced incidence of illness symptoms following competitive events.

– Avoid very prolonged training sessions (>2 h) and excessive periods of intensified training. Adequate recovery is important to avoid overtraining and chronic fatigue. Periodization of training will help to avoid becoming stale. Avoid training monotony by ensuring variation in the day-to-day training load: ensure that a hard training day is followed by a day of lighter training. Monitoring of symptoms of overreaching (mood, feelings of fatigue and muscle soreness) may be helpful [24].

– When training sessions are performed in a fasting or low-glycogen state and without carbohydrate ingestion during exercise, it is likely that a more substantial degree of immune depression will develop [23], especially if this is not the first training session of the day. If this train-low (glycogen) concept is to be applied to maximize training adaptation [25], it should not be done for more than a few days per week or immune function will be compromised.

– The consumption of beverages during exercise not only helps prevent dehydration (which is associated with an increased stress hormone response) but also helps to maintain saliva flow rate during exercise. Saliva contains several proteins with antimicrobial properties including immunoglobulin A, lysozyme and α-amylase. Saliva secretion usually falls during exercise, but regular fluid intake during exercise can prevent this.

– The efficacy of most so-called dietary immunostimulants has not been confirmed. However, there is limited evidence that some flavonoids (e.g. quercetin) or flavonoid-containing beverages (e.g. non-alcoholic beer) can reduce URTI incidence in highly physically active people [26–28]. Some well-controlled studies in athletes have indicated that daily probiotic ingestion results in fewer days of respiratory illness and lower severity of URTI symptoms [29–31], and a recent meta-analysis using data from both athlete and non-athlete studies concluded that there is a likely benefit in reducing URTI incidence [32]. Another potential benefit of probiotics could be a reduced risk of gastrointestinal infections – a particular concern when travelling abroad. The studies to date that have shown reduced URTI incidence in athletes have been mostly limited to *Lactobacillus* species and have used daily doses of ~10^{10} live bacteria. Given that some probiotics appear to provide some benefit, with no evidence of harm and are low cost, there is no reason why athletes should not take probiotics, especially if travelling abroad or illness-prone.

– High daily doses (up to 1,000 mg) of vitamin C are not generally justified, but individuals engaged in intensive training and/or cold environments may gain some benefit according to the latest Cochrane systematic review on vitamin C for preventing the common cold [33].

Table 2. Continued

–	Wear appropriate outdoor clothing in inclement weather and avoid getting cold and wet after exercise.
–	Get adequate sleep (at least 7 h per night is recommended). Missing a single night of sleep has little effect on immune function at rest or after exercise, but recent work indicates that the common cold is more prevalent in those who regularly experience low sleep quantity (<7 h per night) and poor sleep quality (frequent awakenings) [34]. Consider monitoring sleep quantity and quality using small, non-invasive movement sensors.
–	Wear flip-flops or similar footwear when going to the showers, swimming pool and locker rooms in order to avoid dermatological diseases.
–	Keep other life stresses to a minimum. Consulting a sport psychologist may be helpful to find ways to reduce stress and adopt suitable coping behaviors.

vitamin D status may also be helpful [20], and this can be assessed using blood tests to measure the plasma concentration of 25-hydroxy vitamin D.

The strategies described in tables 1 and 2 are designed to limit pathogen transmission and maintain immune competence, respectively, assuming that these symptoms all have an infectious cause. While it is certainly true that symptoms of respiratory illness are commonly reported in athletes and are generally associated with impaired athletic performance, an infectious cause of these symptoms has not always been confirmed. A study that examined the causes of symptoms of respiratory illness in both elite and recreational triathletes and a control group of age-matched sedentary subjects over a 5-month period found that only 11 out of 37 illness episodes had an identifiable infectious cause [6], with rhinovirus being the most commonly identified pathogen. There is now a consensus that airway inflammation may be at least partly responsible for some of the respiratory illness symptoms reported by athletes and probably occurs following airway damage caused by high lung ventilation rates during intensive exercise, particularly when breathing cold, dry or polluted air. Allergy can also trigger an inflammatory response, and subsequent symptoms of respiratory illness are very similar to those caused by infections. A recent study on over 200 runners who participated in the 2010 London marathon found a strong correlation between the prevalence of allergy and post-race reporting of symptoms of upper respiratory illness [21]. Allergy is both treatable and manageable if correctly diagnosed, but until recently has not generally been considered as a cause of respiratory illness by sport physicians. This suggests that screening for common allergens could be a useful addition to the recommended strategies to help minimize respiratory illness episodes in athletes.

Should infection occur, athletes can follow some basic guidelines for exercise during infectious episodes [30] before being referred to a doctor (table 3). These guidelines relate to the illness symptoms that are evident in the athlete and whether these symptoms persist, improve or worsen.

Table 3. Guidelines for training when suffering from URTI in athletes

– First day of illness: Avoid strenuous exercise or competitions when experiencing URTI symptoms like sore throat, coughing, runny or congested nose. Avoid all exercise when experiencing symptoms like muscle/joint pain and headache, fever and generalized feeling of malaise, diarrhea or vomiting.
– Second day: Avoid exercise if fever, diarrhea or vomiting is present or if coughing is increased. If no fever or malaise is present and there is no worsening of 'above the collar' symptoms, undertake light exercise (heart rate <120 beats per min) for 30–45 min (indoors during winter) by yourself.
– Third day: If fever and URTI (or gastrointestinal) symptoms are still present, consult your doctor. If no fever or malaise is present and there is no worsening of initial symptoms, undertake moderate exercise (heart rate <150 beats per min) for 45–60 min, preferably indoors and by yourself.
– Fourth day: If there is no symptom relief, do not try to exercise and pay a visit to your doctor. If this is the first day of improved condition, wait one day without fever and with improvement of URTI or gastrointestinal symptoms before returning to exercise.
– Finally, it is important to stop training and consult your doctor if a new episode with fever occurs or if initial symptoms become worse, coughing persists or breathing problems during exercise occur.

Table 4. Guidelines for returning to training after an episode of URTI in athletes

– Make sure you have had at least one day without fever and with improvement of other illness symptoms before resuming exercise sessions.
– Observe your body's reaction to your first exercise session before beginning a new session.
– Begin with light training and build gradually over several days.
– Observe your tolerance to increased exercise intensity and take a day off training if recovery is less than satisfactory.
– Stop exercise altogether and consult your doctor if there is a recurrence of fever or if initial symptoms become worse, coughing persists or breathing problems during exercise occur.

When recovering from a respiratory illness, it is important to closely observe the individual athlete's symptoms and tolerance to increasing training load. The following guidelines [35] can be given (table 4), but the golden rule must always be to stop training and consult a doctor if symptoms recur.

Conclusions

There is now substantial evidence to support the notion that prolonged strenuous exercise is associated with a transient suppression of immune functions which usually recover within 24 h. However, in situations of intensive training, a lack of sufficient recovery between exercise sessions can lead to chronic depression of immune responses. It has been suggested that such effects on host defense account for the apparent higher incidence of upper respiratory and gastrointestinal illness among highly trained athletes, leading to absence from training and impaired performance. While it is certainly true that symptoms of respiratory and gastrointestinal illness are commonly reported in athletes, an infectious cause of these symptoms, particularly with regard to respiratory illnesses, has not always been confirmed. There are various training, behavioral and nutritional strategies that can help to minimize URTI risk, and these should become part of the athlete's normal routine. A possible concern with intensive exercise training from an early age and over many years is a premature involution of the thymus and alteration of the T cell repertoire which in later life may compromise the ability to respond to new infectious challenges.

Disclosure Statement

M. Gleeson has received funding for research from GlaxoSmithKline, Nestlé, PepsiCo and Yakult.

References

1 Matthews CE, Ockene IS, Freedson PS, et al: Moderate to vigorous physical activity and the risk of upper-respiratory tract infection. Med Sci Sports Exerc 2002;34:1242–1248.

2 Nieman DC, Henson DA, Austin MD, Sha W: Upper respiratory tract infection is reduced in physically fit and active adults. Br J Sports Med 2011;45:987–992.

3 Walsh NP, Gleeson M, Shephard RJ, et al: Position statement part one: immune function and exercise. Exerc Immunol Rev 2011; 17:6–63.

4 Nieman DC, Johanssen LM, Lee JW, Arabatzis K: Infectious episodes in runners before and after the Los Angeles Marathon. J Sports Med Phys Fitness 1990;30:316–328.

5 Peters EM, Bateman ED: Ultramarathon running and upper respiratory tract infections. An epidemiological survey. S Afr Med J 1983; 64:582–584.

6 Spence L, Brown WJ, Pyne DB, et al: Incidence, etiology, and symptomatology of upper respiratory illness in elite athletes. Med Sci Sports Exerc 2007;39:577–586.

7 Gleeson M (ed): Immune Function in Sport and Exercise. Edinburgh, Elsevier, 2005.

8 Alonso JM, Edouard P, Fischetto G, et al: Determination of future prevention strategies in elite track and field: analysis of Daegu 2011 IAAF Championships injuries and illnesses surveillance. Br J Sports Med 2012;46:505–514.

9 Walsh NP, Gleeson M, Pyne DB, et al: Position statement part two: maintaining immune health. Exerc Immunol Rev 2011;17:64–103.

10 Gleeson M, Bishop NC, Oliveira M, et al: Sex differences in immune variables and respiratory infection incidence in an athletic population. Exerc Immunol Rev 2011;17:122–135.

11 Gleeson M: Immune system adaptation in elite athletes. Curr Opin Clin Nutr Metab Care 2006;9:659–665.

12 Bishop NC, Gleeson M: Acute and chronic effects of exercise on markers of mucosal immunity. Front Biosci 2009;14:4444–4456.

13 Neville V, Gleeson M, Folland JP: Salivary IgA as a risk factor for upper respiratory infections in elite professional athletes. Med Sci Sports Exerc 2008;40:1228–1236.

14 Gleeson M, Pyne DB, Austin JP, et al: Epstein-Barr virus reactivation and upper-respiratory illness in elite swimmers. Med Sci Sports Exerc 2002;34:411–417.

15 Prieto A, Knight A, Compton C, et al: Premature immune senescence in elite athletes. J Immunol, in press.

16 Gleeson M, Siegler J, Burke LM, et al: A to Z of nutritional supplements: dietary supplements, sports nutrition foods and ergogenic aids for health and performance – part 31. Br J Sports Med 2012;46:377–378.

17 Costa RJ, Fortes MB, Richardson K, et al: The effects of postexercise feeding on saliva antimicrobial proteins. Int J Sport Nutr Exerc Metab 2012;22:184–191.

18 Costa RJ, Walters R, Bilzon JLJ, Walsh NP: Effects of immediate postexercise carbohydrate ingestion with and without protein on neutrophil degranulation. Int J Sport Nutr Exerc Metab 2011;21:205–213.

19 Fortes MB, Diment BC, Di Felice U, Walsh NP: Dehydration decreases saliva antimicrobial proteins important for mucosal immunity. Appl Physiol Nutr Metab 2012;37:850–859.

20 Larson-Meyer DE, Willis KS: Vitamin D and athletes. Curr Sports Med Rep 2010;9:220–226.

21 Robson-Ansley P, Howatson G, Tallent J, et al: Prevalence of allergy and upper respiratory tract symptoms in runners of the London Marathon. Med Sci Sports Exerc 2012;44:999–1004.

22 Kamen DL, Tangpricha V: Vitamin D and molecular actions on the immune system: modulation of innate and autoimmunity. J Mol Med 2010;88:441–450.

23 Gleeson M: Exercise, nutrition and immunity; in Calder PC, Yaqoob P (eds): Diet, Immunity and Inflammation. Cambridge, Woodhead Publishing, 2013, chapter 26.

24 Meeusen R, Duclos M, Foster C, et al: Prevention, diagnosis and treatment of the overtraining syndrome. Joint consensus statement of the European College of Sport Science (ECSS) and the American College of Sports Medicine (ACSM). Eur J Sport Sci 2013;13:1–24.

25 Hawley JA, Burke LM: Carbohydrate availability and training adaptation: effects on cell metabolism. Exerc Sport Sci Rev 2010;38:152–160.

26 Nieman DC, Henson DA, Gross SJ, et al: Quercetin reduces illness but not immune perturbations after intensive exercise. Med Sci Sports Exerc 2007;39:1561–1569.

27 Heinz SA, Henson DA, Austin MD, et al: Quercetin supplementation and upper respiratory tract infection: a randomized community clinical trial. Pharmacol Res 2010;62:237–242.

28 Scherr J, Nieman DC, Schuster T, et al: Non-alcoholic beer reduces inflammation and incidence of respiratory tract illness. Med Sci Sports Exerc 2012;44:18–26.

29 Cox AJ, Pyne DB, Saunders PU, et al: Oral administration of the probiotic Lactobacillus fermentum VRI-003 and mucosal immunity in endurance athletes. Br J Sports Med 2010;44:222–226.

30 Gleeson M, Bishop NC, Oliveira M, et al: Daily probiotic's *(Lactobacillus casei Shirota)* reduction of infection incidence in athletes. Int J Sport Nutr Exerc Metab 2011;21:55–64.

31 West NP, Pyne DB, Cripps AW, et al: *Lactobacillus fermentum* (PCC(R)) supplementation and gastrointestinal and respiratory-tract illness symptoms: a randomised control trial in athletes. Nutr J 2011;10:30.

32 Hao Q, Lu Z, Dong BR, et al: Probiotics for preventing acute upper respiratory tract infections. Cochrane Database Syst Rev 2011;CD006895.

33 Douglas RM, Hemila H, Chalker E, et al: Vitamin C for preventing and treating the common cold. Cochrane Database Syst Rev 2007;CD000980.

34 Cohen S, Doyle WJ, Alper CM, et al: Sleep habits and susceptibility to the common cold. Arch Intern Med 2009;169:62–67.

35 Ronsen O: Prevention and management of respiratory tract infections in athletes. New Stud Athl 2005;20:49–56.

van Loon LJC, Meeusen R (eds): Limits of Human Endurance.
Nestlé Nutr Inst Workshop Ser, vol 76, pp 51–60, (DOI: 10.1159/000350256)
Nestec Ltd., Vevey/S. Karger AG., Basel, © 2013

Physiological and Performance Adaptations to High-Intensity Interval Training

Martin J. Gibala[a] · Andrew M. Jones[b]

[a]Department of Kinesiology, McMaster University, Hamilton, ON, Canada;
[b]Department of Sport and Health Sciences, University of Exeter, Exeter, UK

Abstract

High-intensity interval training (HIIT) refers to exercise that is characterized by relatively short bursts of vigorous activity, interspersed by periods of rest or low-intensity exercise for recovery. In untrained and recreationally active individuals, short-term HIIT is a potent stimulus to induce physiological remodeling similar to traditional endurance training despite a markedly lower total exercise volume and training time commitment. As little as six sessions of 'all-out' HIIT over 14 days, totaling ~15 min of intense cycle exercise within total training time commitment of ~2.5 h, is sufficient to enhance exercise capacity and improve skeletal muscle oxidative capacity. From an athletic standpoint, HIIT is also an effective strategy to improve performance when supplemented into the already high training volumes of well-trained endurance athletes, although the underlying mechanisms are likely different compared to less trained subjects. Most studies in this regard have examined the effect of replacing a portion (typically ~15–25%) of base/normal training with HIIT (usually 2–3 sessions per week for 4–8 weeks). It has been proposed that a polarized approach to training, in which ~75% of total training volume be performed at low intensities, with 10–15% performed at very high intensities may be the optimal training intensity distribution for elite athletes who compete in intense endurance events.

Copyright © 2013 Nestec Ltd., Vevey/S. Karger AG, Basel

Introduction

High-intensity interval training (HIIT) refers to exercise that is characterized by relatively short bursts of vigorous activity, interspersed by periods of rest or low-intensity exercise for recovery. HIIT is almost infinitely variable, and the specific physiological adaptations induced by this form of training are likely determined by many factors including the mode and precise nature of the exercise stimulus, i.e. the intensity, duration and number of intervals performed, as well as the duration and activity patterns during recovery. In untrained and recreationally active individuals, short-term HIIT is a potent stimulus to induce physiological remodeling similar to traditional endurance training despite a markedly lower total exercise volume and training time commitment [1–3]. These findings are noteworthy from a public health perspective, given that 'lack of time' remains one of the most commonly cited barriers to regular exercise participation [4]. From an athletic standpoint, HIIT is also an effective strategy to improve performance when supplemented into the already high training volumes of well-trained endurance athletes [5–9]. This brief review considers some of the mechanisms responsible for enhanced aerobic energy provision after low-volume HIIT, although this work is based largely on studies conducted on untrained or recreationally active individuals. The other focus is the practical application of HIIT to improve athletic performance, recognizing that the underlying mechanisms are likely different compared to less trained subjects.

Adaptations to Low-Volume HIIT in Untrained and Recreationally Active Individuals

The most common model employed in low-volume HIIT studies has been the Wingate Test, which consists of 30 s of 'all-out' cycling on a specialized ergometer [10]. Mean power output generated during a Wingate Test is very high and typically corresponds to a value that is ~2–3 times greater than achieved at the end of a standard maximal oxygen uptake (VO_2max) test. Wingate-based HIIT typically consists of 4–6 work bouts separated by a few minutes of recovery, for a total of 2–3 min of intense exercise spread over a training session that lasts ~20 min. As little as six sessions of this type of training over 14 days, totaling ~15 min of all-out cycle exercise within total training time commitment of ~2.5 h, is sufficient to dramatically improve exercise capacity in untrained and recreationally active individuals. For example, Burgomaster et al. [11] showed that subjects doubled the length of time that exercise could be maintained at a fixed submaximal workload – from ~26 to 51 min during cycling at 80% of pretraining VO_2max – after only 2 weeks of HIIT. Other work has shown that a similar period of HIIT improved performance during tasks that more closely resemble normal athletic competition, including laboratory time trials that simulated cycling races lasting from ~2 min to ~1 h [2, 12].

With respect to physiological adaptations, as little as 6 sessions of Wingate-based HIIT over 2 weeks is a potent stimulus to enhance skeletal muscle oxidative capacity, as reflected by the maximal activity and/or protein content of mitochondrial enzymes [2, 11]. We have also directly compared responses to 6 weeks of Wingate-based HIIT versus a much higher volume of continuous moderate-intensity endurance training that was designed according to current public health guidelines [1, 13]. These studies revealed similar training-induced improvements in VO_2max and various markers of skeletal muscle and cardiovascular adaptation despite large differences in weekly training volume (~90% lower in the HIIT group) and time commitment (~67% lower in the HIIT group). In addition to an increased skeletal muscle oxidative capacity [1] and enhanced peripheral vascular structure and function [13], other endurance-related adaptations that are apparent after several weeks of Wingate-based HIIT include a reduced rate of glycogen utilization and lactate production during matched-work exercise, an increased capacity for whole-body and skeletal muscle lipid oxidation and increased muscle content of metabolic transport proteins [1, 2, 11, 12].

Some of these physiological adaptations may well have been responsible for the faster O_2 uptake kinetics during exercise reported following HIIT [14, 15]. In the study by Bailey et al. [14], 24 recreationally active subjects were divided into three groups: a control group which completed no additional exercise training; a HIIT group which completed six sessions of 4–7 × 30-second Wingate sprints, and an endurance training group which completed six sessions of work-matched, moderate-intensity cycling. All subjects completed moderate-intensity and high-intensity 'step' exercise transitions before and after the 2-week intervention period. Following HIIT, the phase 2 VO_2 kinetics was significantly speeded by 20–25% for both moderate-intensity and severe-intensity exercise, and the amplitude of the VO_2 slow component, which reflects a progressive loss of metabolic stability during high-intensity exercise, was significantly reduced. Moreover, following HIIT, the time to exhaustion during high-intensity exercise was improved by 53% (from 700 ± 234 to 1,074 ± 431 s). Neither VO_2 kinetics nor performance was significantly altered in the control group or the endurance training group. Interestingly, the improved VO_2 kinetics in the HIIT group was associated with changes in the muscle deoxygenation signal, measured with near infra-red spectroscopy, which suggested that muscle fractional O_2 extraction was enhanced. The improvement in VO_2 kinetics following HIIT likely reflects physiological adaptations to the training which improved muscle blood flow and its distribution as well as muscle metabolic control [16].

Wingate-based training is very potent; however, low-volume HIIT does not have to be 'all out' in order to be effective. Recently, a model was proposed that might be more 'practical', in that it does not require a specialized ergometer and may have wider application to different populations including people at risk for cardiometabolic disorders [17]. The protocol consists of 10×60-second work bouts at a constant-load intensity that elicits ~90% of maximal heart rate, interspersed with 60 s of recovery. The method is still time efficient in that only 10 min of exercise is performed over a 20-min training session. Importantly, the model is also effective at inducing rapid skeletal muscle remodeling towards a more oxidative phenotype [17], similar to previous Wingate-based HIIT studies and high-volume endurance training [1]. We also showed in a small pilot study that the protocol was well tolerated by patients with type 2 diabetes, and 6 sessions over 2 weeks was sufficient to reduce average 24-hour blood glucose concentration, measured via continuous glucose monitoring under standardized diet but otherwise free-living conditions [18]. These beneficial adaptations were realized even though the weekly training time commitment was much lower than common public health guidelines that generally call for at least 150 min of moderate to vigorous exercise per week to promote health.

Recently, Gunnarsson and Bangsbo [19] investigated the physiological effect of an alteration from standard endurance training to interval training on indicators of cardiovascular health, muscle metabolism, VO_2max and performance in moderately trained runners. The subjects were divided into a high-intensity training group and a control group which continued with normal training. For a 7-week intervention period, the interval training group replaced all training sessions with low-, moderate-, and high-speed running (<30, <60, and >90% of maximal intensity) for 30, 20, and 10 s, respectively, in three or four 5-min blocks interspersed by 2 min of recovery. In this way, training volume was reduced from approximately 30 to 14 km of running per week. After the intervention period, VO_2max in the interval training group was increased by 4%, and performance in a 1,500-meter and a 5-km run improved significantly (by 21 and 48 s, respectively). Moreover, systolic blood pressure was reduced and total and low-density lipoprotein cholesterol were significantly lower. No alterations were observed in CON across the intervention period. Interestingly, muscle membrane proteins and enzyme activity did not change in either of the groups. This study reveals another type of HIIT that can improve both the cardiovascular health profile and exercise performance. Specifically, interval training involving 10-second near-maximal bouts can improve performance despite a ~50% reduction in training volume.

Anecdotally, patients prefer to complete HIIT sessions than longer bouts of low-intensity exercise. Because HIIT accelerates the adaptation to training, this may provide patient or sedentary populations of low fitness with early encouragement which may translate into improved adherence to a longer-term training program. HIIT may be especially beneficial early in a training intervention in such populations, and may be supplemented with traditional aerobic training later on to maximize training adaptations. Another advantage of HIIT is that, unlike traditional endurance training, it provides almost infinite variety, with the number, duration and intensity of each of the work bouts being adjustable, along with the duration and intensity of the recovery intervals. This may enable interest to be maintained over the longer-term. In summary, in previously untrained or recreationally active individuals, low-volume HIIT is a time-efficient strategy to rapidly improve exercise capacity and stimulate numerous physiological adaptations that are normally associated with traditional endurance training.

It is interesting to consider the adaptations to HIIT in light of the determinants of endurance performance put forward in the well-established model of Ed Coyle [20]. This model proposes that endurance performance is chiefly a function of the VO_2max, efficiency during submaximal exercise (which is more commonly termed economy during running), and the fractional utilization of the VO_2max. The former is important because the performance VO_2 clearly cannot exceed the VO_2max; efficiency is important because it determines the performance speed corresponding to a given VO_2, and fractional utilization is important because it dictates the VO_2 that can be sustained for a given distance or exercise duration. While longer term HIIT may invoke central cardiovascular adaptations which underpin an increased VO_2max, it appears, at least in the short term, that HIIT mainly stimulates peripheral muscle metabolic adaptations [3]. In terms of Coyle's model [20], HIIT-induced improvements in substrate utilization and oxidative energy turnover may therefore enhance endurance capacity by increasing the fractional utilization of the VO_2max. Also, although not reported explicitly, we have noticed in several studies that even short-term HIIT consistently results in a small but significant reduction in the O_2 cost of submaximal exercise, which may be evidence of improved efficiency.

Effect of HIIT in Highly Trained Individuals

In comparison to untrained and recreationally active subjects, much less is known about the response of highly trained individuals to HIIT. Although typically an integral component of training programs for the enhancement of athletic performance, research into the unique effects of HIIT on the performance of well-trained individuals is sparse [5]. As noted by Hawley et al. [5], there are various reasons for this including the fact that sports scientists have found it difficult to persuade elite athletes to experiment with their training regimes. Indeed, scientists themselves have urged caution in giving training recommendations to athletes and coaches based on the relatively limited literature available [21]. Nonetheless, there is evidence to suggest that inserting a relatively short period of HIIT into the already high training volumes of well-trained athletes can further enhance performance [5–9]. Most studies in this regard have examined the effect of replacing a portion (typically ~15–25%) of base/normal training with HIIT (usually 2–3 sessions per week for 4–8 weeks). Improvements in performance with this approach have generally been interpreted to be due to the inclusion of the HIIT, although it is possible that the reduced training volume per se also contributes to some degree. The precise nature of the HIIT stimulus has varied from repeated intervals lasting up to 5 min at an intensity eliciting ~80% VO_2max to 30-second efforts at an all-out pace or power outputs corresponding to ≥175% of VO_2max.

One of the first studies to demonstrate the beneficial effect of HIIT on performance in trained subjects was conducted by Acevedo and Goldfarb [22]. These authors examined the effect of 8 weeks of increased training intensity in 7 competitive male distance runners. Training intensity was increased on 3 days per week by having subjects perform intervals at 90–95% of maximal heart rate or Fartlek style workouts, whereas they maintained their habitual continuous runs on the other days of the week. 10-km race time improved after the intervention by over 1 min from 35:27 to 34:24, despite no change in VO_2max. Other investigators have subsequently reported performance improvements when trained runners reduced their total training volume but increased intensity through the addition of brief all-out HIIT efforts [23]. For a 6- to 9-week period, Bangsbo et al. [23] assigned runners to a group that replaced approximately one quarter of their normal training volume with 12 × 30-second all-out sprint runs 3–4 times per week, or a group that continued with their normal endurance training (~55 km/week). VO_2max was not altered; however, the HIIT intervention improved 3 km (from 10.4 to 10.1 min) and 10 km run time (from 37.3 to 36.3 min), whereas the control group showed no change in performance. Similarly, Smith et al. [24] reported that trained runners who completed 4 weeks of HIIT (consisting of 6 × ~2 min at VO_2max running speed, 2×/week) improved 3-km run performance compared to a group that continued with their normal training.

Researchers in South Africa conducted a series of studies in the 1990s that examined the effect of HIIT in well-trained competitive cyclists [25–28]. The subjects in these studies were all men with a training history of at least 3–4 years who were cycling at ~300 km/week, but had not undertaken any interval training for several months before investigation. They typically presented with VO_2max values ≥65 ml/kg per min and peak sustained power outputs >400 W, confirming their highly trained state [reviewed in 5]. Lindsay et al. [25] examined the effect of replacing 15% of the cyclists' normal base training with interval training, which consisted of 6–8 repetitions × 5 min at an intensity that elicited 80% of each subject's peak power output (PPO), interspersed with 60 s of recovery. After 6 sessions of HIIT over a 4 weeks' period, the cyclists improved their peak power and speed during a 40-km time trial that translated into improved performance (56.4 vs. 54.4 min). Stepto et al. [26] investigated the effect of varying the intensity and duration of a 3-week (6 sessions) HIIT stimulus on 40-km time trial performance. Twenty well-trained cyclists were randomly assigned to one of five types of interval-training session: 12 × 30 s at 175% PPO, 12 × 60 s at 100% PPO, 12 × 2 min at 90% PPO, 8 × 4 min at 85% PPO, or 4 × 8 min at 80% PPO. As the authors hypothesized, training sessions that employed work bouts that were closely matched to race pace (8 × 4 min at 85% PPO) significantly enhanced performance (2.8%, 95% CI: 4.3–1.3%). Somewhat surprisingly, the short duration, supra-maximal work bouts (12 × 30 s at 175% of PPO) were just as effective in improving performance (2.4%, 95% CI: 4.0–0.7%), whereas the other interval protocols did not produce statistically significant improvements in performance. However, the sample size in each group was small (n = 4), and Laursen et al. [29] have subsequently reported that 40-km time trial performance is improved in trained cyclists after a 4-week HIIT protocol that consists of 8 × ~2.5 bouts per session at an intensity equivalent to 100% PPO.

The mechanisms responsible for the observed performance improvements after HIIT in highly trained individuals are likely different compared to less trained subjects. Whereas rapid increases in skeletal muscle oxidative capacity are observed after a short period of low-volume HIIT in untrained and recreationally active subjects [2, 11, 12, 17], several weeks of HIIT does not further increase the maximal activity of mitochondrial enzymes in highly trained individuals [27, 28]. HIIT has been reported to improve skeletal muscle buffering capacity in highly trained subjects, and it has also been suggested that training-induced changes in Na^+/K^+ pump activity may help to preserve cell excitability and force production, thereby delay fatigue development during intense exercise [8].

It has been proposed that a polarized approach to training, in which ~75% of total training volume be performed at low intensities, with 10–15% performed at very high intensities may be the optimal training intensity distribution for elite athletes who compete in intense endurance events [9]. While it is clear that many athletes do adopt this approach, there are also examples of highly accomplished athletes who complete their continuous 'steady-state' training at relatively high intensities and who include sustained 'tempo' training sessions in their weekly program [30]. It would therefore seem appropriate for athletes to use a variety of approaches, in a carefully balanced selection of training sessions across the intensity-duration continuum, to optimize the stimuli for physiological adaptation. By activating both the adenosine monophosphate kinase and calcium-calmodulin kinase signaling pathways, this may provide a potent stimulus to the so-called 'master switch', peroxisome proliferator-activated receptor-g coactivator-1a, which in turn may lead to a variety of adaptations likely to enhance endurance exercise performance.

Although inserting a relatively short period of HIIT into the high training volumes of well-trained athletes can further enhance performance [5–9], it is unlikely that this approach is sustainable in the longer-term. It is feasible that such training, if undertaken continuously, could result in overtraining. Therefore, it is recommended that HIIT be used periodically as an additional stimulus to adaptation, perhaps every 8–10 weeks and/or in the taper period prior to a major competition.

Little is known regarding the potential for nutrition or other interventions to augment physiological and performance effects of HIIT in elite athletes. For example, it is feasible that performing HIIT in hypoxia might further increase the signaling which results in enhanced angiogenesis or mitochondrial biogenesis. However, one study found short-term hypoxic exposure did not elicit a greater increase in performance or hematological modifications compared to HIIT alone in well-trained cyclists and triathletes [31]. Several nutritional ergogenic aids including caffeine, creatine, nitrate, sodium bicarbonate and β-alanine, alone or in combination, during HIIT could theoretically facilitate training quality acutely and thus result in an improved training outcome. In this regard, Edge et al. [32] reported that subjects who ingested sodium bicarbonate over an 8-week high-intensity intermittent cycle training program, matched for total volume, experienced greater improvements in time trial performance compared to a placebo group. Another interesting question is whether the potent effects of HIIT on physiological adaptations and performance are linked more to the absolute intensity achieved in each of the work bouts or simply to the repeated transient metabolic challenges inherent to interval training. The absolute intensity of the work bout will dictate the motor unit recruitment profile. It is possible that HIIT is effective, at least in part, because it activates and thus enhances the metabolic profile of the type 2 fibers that are positioned higher in the recruitment hierarchy. Alternatively or additionally, the repeated metabolic perturbations (rapid changes in the concentrations of ATP, ADP, Pi, PCr, etc.) in the abrupt transitions from rest to exercise may be important in evoking the cellular adaptations known to occur following HIIT. Further research is required to investigate these important questions.

Conclusion

In untrained and recreationally active individuals, short-term HIIT is a potent stimulus to induce physiological adaptations similar to traditional endurance training. As little as six sessions of 'all-out' HIIT over 14 days, totaling ~15 min of intense cycle exercise, is sufficient to enhance skeletal muscle oxidative capacity and exercise endurance. HIIT is also an effective strategy to improve performance when it replaces some of the high training volume in the programs of well-trained endurance athletes, although the specific mechanisms may be different compared to less trained individuals. It has been proposed that a polarized approach to training, in which ~75% of total training volume be performed at low intensities, with 10–15% performed at very high intensities may be the optimal training intensity distribution for elite athletes who compete in intense endurance events.

Disclosure Statement

The authors declare that no financial or other conflict of interest exists in relation to the content of the chapter.

References

1 Burgomaster KA, Howarth KR, Phillips SM, et al: Similar metabolic adaptations during exercise after low volume sprint interval and traditional endurance training in humans. J Physiol 2008;586:151–160.

2 Gibala MJ, Little JP, van Essen M, et al: Short-term sprint interval versus traditional endurance training: similar initial adaptations in human skeletal muscle and exercise performance. J Physiol 2006;575: 901–911.

3 Gibala MJ, Little JP, Macdonald MJ, Hawley JA: Physiological adaptations to low-volume, high-intensity interval training in health and disease. J Physiol 2012;590:1077–1084.

4 Stutts WC: Physical activity determinants in adults. Perceived benefits, barriers, and self efficacy. AAOHN J 2002;50:499–507.

5 Hawley JA, Myburgh KH, Noakes TD, Dennis SC: Training techniques to improve fatigue resistance and enhance endurance performance. J Sports Sci 1997;15:25–33.

6 Iaia FM, Bangsbo J: Speed endurance training is a powerful stimulus for physiological adaptations and performance improvements of athletes. Scand J Med Sci Sports 2010; 20(suppl 2):11–23.

7 Kubukeli ZN, Noakes TD, Dennis SC: Training techniques to improve endurance exercise performances. Sports Med 2002;32:489–509.

8 Laursen PB, Jenkins DG: The scientific basis for high-intensity interval training: optimising training programmes and maximising performance in highly trained endurance athletes. Sports Med 2002;32:53–73.

9 Laursen PB: Training for intense exercise performance: high-intensity or high-volume training? Scand J Med Sci Sports 2010; 20(suppl 2):1–10.

10 Bar-Or O: The Wingate anaerobic test. An update on methodology, reliability and validity. Sports Med 1987;4:381–394.

11 Burgomaster KA, Hughes SC, Heigenhauser GJ, et al: Six sessions of sprint interval training increases muscle oxidative potential and cycle endurance capacity in humans. J Appl Physiol 2005;98:1985–1990.

12 Burgomaster KA, Heigenhauser GJ, Gibala MJ: Effect of short-term sprint interval training on human skeletal muscle carbohydrate metabolism during exercise and time-trial performance. J Appl Physiol 2006;100:2041–2047.

13 Rakobowchuk M, Tanguay S, Burgomaster KA, et al: Sprint interval and traditional endurance training induce similar improvements in peripheral arterial stiffness and flow-mediated dilation in healthy humans. Am J Physiol Regul Integr Comp Physiol 2008;295:R236–R242.

14 Bailey SJ, Wilkerson DP, Dimenna FJ, Jones AM: Influence of repeated sprint training on pulmonary O_2 uptake and muscle deoxygenation kinetics in humans. J Appl Physiol 2009;106:1875–1887.

15 McKay BR, Paterson DH, Kowalchuk JM: Effect of short-term high-intensity interval training vs. continuous training on O_2 uptake kinetics, muscle deoxygenation, and exercise performance. J Appl Physiol 2009; 107:128–138.

16 Jones AM, Grassi B, Christensen PM, et al: Slow component of VO_2 kinetics: mechanistic bases and practical applications. Med Sci Sports Exerc 2011;43:2046–2062.

17 Little JP, Safdar A, Wilkin GP, et al: A practical model of low-volume high-intensity interval training induces mitochondrial biogenesis in human skeletal muscle: potential mechanisms. J Physiol 2010;588:1011–1022.

18 Little JP, Gillen JB, Percival ME, et al: Low-volume high-intensity interval training reduces hyperglycemia and increases muscle mitochondrial capacity in patients with type 2 diabetes. J Appl Physiol 2011;111:1554–1560.

19 Gunnarsson TP, Bangsbo J: The 10-20-30 training concept improves performance and health profile in moderately trained runners. J Appl Physiol 2012;113:16–24.

20 Coyle EF: Integration of the physiological factors determining endurance performance ability. Exerc Sport Sci Rev 1995;23:25–63.

21 Midgley AW, McNaughton LR, Jones AM: Training to enhance the physiological determinants of long-distance running performance: can valid recommendations be given to runners and coaches based on current scientific knowledge? Sports Med 2007;37:857–880.

22 Acevedo EO, Goldfarb AH: Increased training intensity effects on plasma lactate, ventilatory threshold, and endurance. Med Sci Sports Exerc 1989;21:563–568.

23 Bangsbo J, Gunnarsson TP, Wendell J, et al: Reduced volume and increased training intensity elevate muscle Na+-K+ pump alpha2-subunit expression as well as short- and long-term work capacity in humans. J Appl Physiol 2009;107:1771–1780.

24 Smith TP, Coombes JS, Geraghty DP: Optimising high-intensity treadmill training using the running speed at maximal O_2 uptake and the time for which this can be maintained. Eur J Appl Physiol 2003;89:337–343.

25 Lindsay FH, Hawley JA, Myburgh KH, et al: Improved athletic performance in highly trained cyclists after interval training. Med Sci Sports Exerc 1996;28:1427–1434.

26 Stepto NK, Hawley JA, Dennis SC, Hopkins WG: Effects of different interval-training programs on cycling time-trial performance. Med Sci Sports Exerc 1999;31:736–741.

27 Westgarth-Taylor C, Hawley JA, Rickard S, et al: Metabolic and performance adaptations to interval training in endurance-trained cyclists. Eur J Appl Physiol Occup Physiol 1997; 75:298–304.

28 Weston AR, Myburgh KH, Lindsay FH, et al: Skeletal muscle buffering capacity and endurance performance after high-intensity interval training by well-trained cyclists. Eur J Appl Physiol Occup Physiol 1997;75:7–13.

29 Laursen PB, Shing CM, Peake JM, et al: Interval training program optimization in highly trained endurance cyclists. Med Sci Sports Exerc 2002;34:1801–1807.

30 Jones AM: The physiology of the world record holder for the women's marathon. Int J Sports Sci Coach 2006;1:101–116.

31 Roels B, Millet GP, Marcoux CJ, et al: Effects of hypoxic interval training on cycling performance. Med Sci Sports Exerc 2005;37: 138–146.

32 Edge J, Bishop D, Goodman C: Effects of chronic NaHCO3 ingestion during interval training on changes to muscle buffer capacity, metabolism, and short-term endurance performance. J Appl Physiol 2006;101:918–925.

van Loon LJC, Meeusen R (eds): Limits of Human Endurance.
Nestlé Nutr Inst Workshop Ser, vol 76, pp 61–71, (DOI: 10.1159/000350258)
Nestec Ltd., Vevey/S. Karger AG., Basel, © 2013

Effect of β-Alanine Supplementation on High-Intensity Exercise Performance

Roger C. Harris[a] · Trent Stellingwerff[b]

[a] Junipa Ltd., Newmarket, UK; [b] Canadian Sports Centre-Pacific, Pacific Institute for Sport Excellence, Victoria, BC, Canada

Abstract

Carnosine is a dipeptide of β-alanine and L-histidine found in high concentrations in skeletal muscle. Combined with β-alanine, the pKa of the histidine imidazole ring is raised to ~6.8, placing it within the muscle intracellular pH high-intensity exercise transit range. Combination with β-alanine renders the dipeptide inert to intracellular enzymic hydrolysis and blocks the histidinyl residue from participation in proteogenesis, thus making it an ideal, stable intracellular buffer. For vegetarians, synthesis is limited by β-alanine availability; for meat-eaters, hepatic synthesis is supplemented with β-alanine from the hydrolysis of dietary carnosine. Direct oral β-alanine supplementation will compensate for low meat and fish intake, significantly raising the muscle carnosine concentration. This is best achieved with a sustained-release formulation of β-alanine to avoid paresthesia symptoms and decreasing urinary spillover. In humans, increased levels of carnosine through β-alanine supplementation have been shown to increase exercise capacity and performance of several types, particularly where the high-intensity exercise range is 1–4 min. β-Alanine supplementation is used by athletes competing in high-intensity track and field cycling, rowing, swimming events and other competitions.

Introduction

β-Alanine is found in muscle in combination with L-histidine forming the dipeptide carnosine (β-alanyl-L-histidine, abbreviated in the context of muscle as M-Carn). Carnosine is a member of a family of three related histidine-containing dipeptides (HCD), the others being anserine [β-alanyl-L-(1-methyl)-histidine] and balenine [β-alanyl-L-(3-methyl)-histidine] [1, 2]. However, carnosine is the only HCD present in human muscle [e.g. m. vastus lateralis, the molar concentration of M-Carn is 4–20 mM (12–60 mmol·kg^{-1} dry muscle)], making it one of most abundant small molecular weight compounds present in resting muscle after phosphorylcreatine (PCr), creatine and ATP. Factors determining the concentration of M-Carn in humans include muscle fiber composition, with a 1.3–2 times higher concentration in fast type 2 compared to type 1 muscle fibers [3–5] and dietary intake of β-alanine [6, 7]. Age and sex may also influence the carnosine content in muscle [7, 8], with postpubertal males having significantly greater carnosine content than females throughout life, and both males and females featuring a steady decline after their mid-twenties [8]. Still, the evidence for this is somewhat tenuous as the changes reported could be secondary to changes in fiber composition (including changes in mean fiber area) and diet. Only one study, Suzuki et al. [9], has reported an effect of training; in this case, a doubling in M-Carn over 8 weeks of training involving a total training time of only 14 min. Conversely, other studies using 4–16 weeks' intensive sprint training [4, 10] and 12 weeks' whole body training [11] have shown no effects on M-Carn. Cross-sectional data of athletes who undertake chronic training have been associated with higher than normal levels of baseline M-Carn [12, 13], although again this may be secondary to changes in fiber composition (and mean fiber area), diet and/or exogenous hormone supplementation (Tallon et al. [12] studied body builders some of whom were known to have supplemented with testosterone). Taken together, it appears that training status plays a minor role in muscle carnosine content, with fiber type composition, dietary carnosine or β-alanine intake and possibly sex hormones being the main determinates of M-Carn.

M-Carn as Buffer of H$^+$ during High-Intensity Exercise

Glycolysis results in the formation of two carboxylic acid groups from the oxidation of neutral hydroxyl groups within each glucose or glycosyl (from glycogen) unit metabolized. Both groups are fully dissociated over the physiological pH range, with a high proportion accumulated as lactate anions (Lac$^-$) and hydrogen cations (H$^+$) during high-intensity exercise (HIE). Lac$^-$ production accounts for the generation of 94% of the H$^+$ produced in skeletal muscle during HIE, causing a decline in intracellular pH (pHi) from ~7.0 at rest to 6.0 in extremis [14]. H$^+$ accumulation may contribute to fatigue by interfering with several metabolic processes affecting force production; the accumulation of H$^+$ disrupts the recovery of PCr compromising its role in the maintenance of [ADP] homeostasis [15] and may disrupt functioning of the muscle contractile machinery [16]. Stabilization of muscle pHi is achieved through export of H$^+$ and in the short term by intracellular physicochemical buffers.

To be effective, a buffer needs to be present in high concentrations and to have a pKa within the exercise pHi transit range (~6.0–7.0). M-Carn satisfies both; occurring in the millimolar range, while the imidazole ring of the histidine residue exhibits a pKa of ~6.8. Other potential muscle buffers include proteins, inorganic and organic phosphates, and bicarbonate present in cells at the start of contraction. The contribution of proteins is limited to their histidine contents; phosphates include both inorganic and organic phosphates. PCr, one of the largest metabolic pools of phosphate has a pKa of 4.58, and thus does not directly contribute to buffering [14]. However, with the start of exercise, decline in the PCr pool, matched by increases in the concentration of inorganic and organic phosphates, will raise the physicochemical buffering capacity of muscle.

The combination of β-alanine with histidine raises the pKa of the imidazole ring to ~6.8, improving its effectiveness in buffering H$^+$ over the exercise pHi transit range. Combination with β-alanine also renders the histidine inert to participation in proteogenesis, enabling high concentrations to be accumulated in muscle cells. This affords a more efficient means to vary the intracellular physicochemical buffering capacity than by alteration of the protein content, where histidine is only 1 of 20 amino acids.

Other Physiological Roles of M-Carn

Other physiological roles have been ascribed to M-Carn including protection of proteins against glycation by acting as a sacrificial peptide, the prevention of protein-protein cross-links through reactions with protein-carbonyl groups, acting as an antioxidant and increasing calcium sensitivity in muscle fibers augmenting force production. Interestingly, Dutka and Lamb [17] and Dutka et al. [18] have recently shown an increase in Ca^{2+} ion sensitivity with increased M-Carn (in rodents and humans) using an in vivo/in vitro preparation with E-C coupling and suggested that higher concentrations of M-Carn could, by this mechanism, delay the onset of fatigue. However, it is by no means certain that Ca^{2+} ion sensitivity, and changes in this, are factors integral to fatigue in whole body exercise.

Regulation of M-Carn by β-Alanine

Carnosine in muscle is synthesized in situ by the action of carnosine synthase (CS):

$$\text{ATP} + \text{L-histidine} + \beta\text{-alanine} \xrightarrow{\text{CS}} \text{AMP} + \text{diphosphate} + \text{carnosine}$$

Synthesis is limited by the β-alanine concentration compared to its Km (1.0–2.3 mM) for CS [2, 19]. In contrast, histidine is present in much higher concentrations in muscle and has a much lower Km (16.8 μM). β-Alanine is synthesized in the liver before being transported to muscle. This may be augmented by β-alanine from the ingestion and hydrolysis of carnosine in muscle meat [20]. The transport of β-alanine into muscle is mediated by a specific β-amino acid transport protein (PEPT2/SLC15A2) that requires both Na$^+$ and Cl$^-$ [21].

In vegetarians, M-Carn is limited by hepatic β-alanine synthesis resulting in low M-Carn compared to omnivores [6, 7]. For omnivores hepatic β-alanine synthesis is augmented by dietary carnosine consumption, resulting in M-Carn levels twice as great as vegetarians [6]. Therefore, it could be hypothesized that the supplementation of β-alanine would increase M-Carn. Indeed, when multiple daily doses of 800 mg (~5.2 g/day) were given over 4 weeks, a mean increase in M-Carn in m. vastus lateralis of 60% was recorded [20]. Extended to 10 weeks, the increase was 80% with absolute values now close to 40 mmol·kg^{-1}·dm^3. The single maximal bolus given was 800 mg (~10 mg·kg^{-1} bodyweight) in order to avoid symptoms of paresthesia, and is equivalent to the β-alanine available from the ingestion of 150 g of chicken breast meat. A maximum of 8 such doses was given per day without any negative effects on clinical chemistry or ECG. Supplementation with an isomolar dose of L-carnosine (13 g/day) resulted in the same M-Carn increases over 4 weeks, showing no additional effect of the histidine also released on hydrolysis [20]. With curtailment of supplementation, M-Carn returns to the pre-supplementation level with an estimated t$_{1/2}$ of 5–9 weeks [5, 22].

Single doses of β-alanine in excess of 10 mg·kg^{-1} bodyweight, or the equivalent molar dose of L-carnosine, administered in solution as a drink or in gelatin capsules cause symptoms of flushing together with a prickly sensation [20]. Symptoms last 15–60 min, and in terms of severity appear dose dependent [23] being absent or very mild at 10 mg·kg^{-1} bodyweight, but severe/uncomfortable at 40 mg·kg^{-1} bodyweight. Possible mechanisms include activation of the Mrg (mas-related gene) family of G protein-coupled receptors [24]. MrgD-containing dorsal route ganglia neurons terminate in the skin and participate in the modulation of neuropathic pain. Recent studies have used a sustained release (SR) formulation (CarnoSyn™, from Natural Alternatives International, San Marcos, Calif., available to the public as High Intensity™, from Power Bar, Florham Park, N.J., USA) enabling two 800 mg SR tablets to be given simultaneously without symptoms of paresthesia [5, 23, 25–28]. For a full review on the delivery and dosing of β-alanine to augment M-Carn refer to Stellingwerff et al. [19].

Ergogenic Effect of Raised M-Carn

In a recent meta-analysis by Hobson et al. [29], 15 published peer-reviewed studies were assessed, from which it was concluded that in exercise tests lasting 60–240 s performance was improved (p = 0.001) as was exercise of >240 s (p = 0.046). There was no benefit of β-alanine supplementation on sprint exercise lasting <60 s (p = 0.312), consistent with the mechanism for the improvement in performance being linked to an increase in H^+ buffering capacity, as opposed to an effect of increased Ca^{2+} ion sensitivity on E-C coupling. In this meta-analysis [29], the median effect of β-alanine supplementation on exercise >60 s was a 2.85% (range –0.37 to 10.49%) improvement in exercise capacity. Hill et al. [3] using a cycle exercise capacity test performed at 110% of maximum power output ($CCT_{110\%}$) and with an expected endurance time of 150 s, showed ~60% increase in M-Carn with 4-week supplementation and an 11.8% improvement in time to exhaustion. This was subsequently repeated by Sale et al. [30], using the same exercise protocol, when an increase of 12.1% in endurance time to exhaustion was recorded.

Three studies have shown a positive correlation between improvements in exercise performance with increases in M-Carn. The exercise modalities included cycling with an expected pre-supplementation endurance time of 150 s [3, 30], rowing over a distance of 2,000 m [31], and, time to exhaustion in a constant-load submaximal test and incremental test in 60- to 80-year-old subjects [26]. The demonstration of a positive cause and effect dose-response relationship between increased M-Carn and performance in these 3 studies is almost unique in studies of dietary ergogenic supplements.

A positive effect of supplementation on isometric endurance of the knee extensors contracting at 45% of maximal voluntary isometric contraction (MVIC) force has recently been reported by Sale et al. [32]. As the circulation to the contracting muscles is largely occluded at 45% MVIC, Lac^- and H^+ loss from the contracting muscle is minimal. Endurance time after 4 weeks of β-alanine supplementation at 6.4 g·day^{-1} was increased by 9.7 s with the estimated increase in

H^+ production matched closely to the estimated increase in H^+ buffering capacity. Whilst isometric exercise is involved in a number of sports, it is more commonly encountered in everyday manual activities involving the lifting and carrying of heavy weights.

Effect on Maximal/Supramaximal Exercise

Since the meta-analysis by Hobson et al. [29], 3 further studies have been published on the effects of supplementation on maximal/supramaximal exercise. Saunders et al. [27] showed no effect on repeated sprint ability using the Loughborough Intermittent Shuttle Test. Although over a longer duration than the 60 s limit suggested by Hobson et al. [29], but still within the category of supramaximal sprint exercise, Jagim et al. [33] showed no effect of β-alanine supplementation on sprint exercise at 115% (lasting ~140–165 s) and 140% VO_2max (lasting ~65–75 s). From these it would seem that supplementation has little effect on HIE of short duration exercise performance (<60 s). However, van Thienen et al. [34] observed a significant performance benefit of β-alanine supplementation on a 30 s cycle sprint following a 110 min submaximal simulated cycle race and 10 min time trial. Under these conditions, the sprint exercise would have begun after muscle pHi had been lowered, and this may explain why supplementation was effective in this case. Similarly, a significant effect of β-alanine supplementation was recorded by Saunders et al. [28] for the YoYo protocol (test of repeated sprints), which is considered highly relevant to team sports such as football, rugby and hockey. In this study, amateur football players undertook repeated bouts of 2 × 20-meter runs against a target time, with 10 s active recovery between bouts. Sprint bouts were maintained until subjects failed to reach the finish line within the allotted time on two consecutive occasions; the total distance covered being used to define performance. Subjects were supplemented with 3.2 g·d^{-1} β-alanine (CarnoSyn SR) tablets for 12 weeks or placebo. β-Alanine supplementation resulted in a significant increase (34%) in total sprint distance covered during the YoYo test [28].

Effect on Longer Duration Submaximal Exercise

Hobson et al. [29] concluded that β-alanine supplementation had a highly significant effect on exercise of >60 s duration. Their conclusion was based on the results from 13 studies. Included in these were 4 studies which examined the effect of supplementation on the physical working capacity at the neuromuscular fatigue threshold [35, 36]. These indicated that supplementation may exhibit effects long before attainment of fatigue, as shown by delayed changes in EMG denoting the neuromuscular fatigue threshold, and leading to increases in the physical working capacity. Such effects were observed in both the young and elderly. Supplemented with β-alanine for 90 days at 2.4 g·d^{-1}, 12 elderly (aged 55–92 years) men and women showed a 29% increase in the physical working capacity at the neuromuscular fatigue threshold, whereas comparable subjects treated with placebo showed no change during the same period [36].

Proof of the effectiveness of dietary β-alanine on M-Carn in the elderly has recently been provided by del Favero et al. [26] using ^{1}H-MRS. Twelve subjects within the age range 60–80 years, supplemented with (2 × 800 mg) × 2·day^{-1} CarnoSyn SR tablets, showed a mean increase of 85% in M-Carn in m. gastrocnemius. Times to exhaustion in a constant-load submaximal test and an incremental test were positively correlated with the increase in M-Carn. It was concluded by the authors that maintaining a high M-Carn could be beneficial in both the immediate and longer term, especially if this encourages subjects to maintain a more active lifestyle and/or increases autonomy in the elderly.

As yet, few studies have been undertaken on the benefits of β-alanine in specific sports, or using exercise models relevant to specific sports, both in elite trained and untrained subjects. In the study by Hill et al. [3], subjects supplemented with β-alanine for 4 and 10 weeks showed a 13 and 16.2% increase in total work done in a cycle capacity test performed at a constant load (CCT$_{110\%}$), mirroring increases of 58.8 and 80.1% in M-Carn in m. vastus lateralis. Confirmation of the results was subsequently provided by Sale et al. [25]. In the study by van Thienen et al. [34], there was no effect of β-alanine on power output in a 10-min time trial undertaken immediately at the end of a simulated 110-min race. However, as noted, peak power output in a 30-second sprint after this was significantly increased by 11% with β-alanine supplementation.

In an examination of the changes in blood pH and oxygen uptake kinetics with 6-min HIE, Baguet et al. [37] observed that exercise-induced acidosis was significantly reduced following β-alanine supplementation compared to placebo without affecting blood lactate. Further, the time delay of the fast component (Td$_1$) of oxygen uptake kinetics was significantly reduced following β-alanine supplementation, although this did not lead to a reduction in oxygen deficit. The parameters of the slow component did not differ between groups. The authors concluded the increase in M-Carn with β-alanine supplementation was effective in attenuating the fall in blood pH during such exercise. Previously, Stout et al. [35] had observed an increase in the ventilatory threshold in female subjects

Table 1. Events at 2012 London Olympics having exercise durations which suggest a potential benefit from supplementation with β-alanine

Discipline	Event	Time, min:s	
		men	women
Track and field	400 m	43.94	49.55
	800 m	1:40.91	1:56.19
	1,500 m	3:34.08	4:10.23
	4 × 400 m	2:56.72	3:16.87
	400 m hurdles	47.63	52.70
Canoeing	K1 500 m	no event	1:51.456
	K2 500 m	no event	1:42.213
	K4 500 m	no event	1:30.827
	K1 1,000 m	3:26.462	no event
	K2 1,000 m	3:09.646	no event
	K4 1,000 m	2:55.085	no event
	C1 1,000 m	3:47.176	no event
	C2 1,000 m	3:33.804	no event
Cycling	3,000 m team pursuit	no event	3:14.051
	4,000 m team pursuit	3:51.659	no event
Rowing (2,000 m)	pair	6:16.65	7:27.13
	four	6:03.97	no event
	lightweight four	6:01.84	no event
	eight	5:48.75	6:10.59
	single sculls	6:57.82	7:54.37
	double sculls	6:31.67	6:55.82
	lightweight double sculls	6:37.17	7:09.30
	quadruple sculls	5:42.48	6:35.93
Swimming	100 m breaststroke	58.46	1:05.47
	100 m backstroke	52.16	58.33
	100 m butterfly	51.21	55.98
	100 m freestyle	47.52	53.00
	200 m breaststroke	2:07.28	2:19.59
	200 m backstroke	1:53.41	2:04.06
	200 m butterfly	1:52.96	2:04.06
	200 m freestyle	1:43.14	1:53.61
	400 m freestyle	3:40.14	4:01.45
	200 m individual medley	1:54.27	2:07.57
	400 m individual medley	4:05.18	4:28.43
	4 × 100 m medley relay	3:29.35	3:52.05
	4 × 100 m freestyle relay	3:09.93	3:33.15
	4 × 200 m freestyle relay	6:59.70	7:42.92

performing a continuous incremental cycle test after 28 days of β-alanine, a result which equally could be explained by an attenuation of the fall in blood pH.

Also of interest to competitive sport, Baguet et al. [31] reported a strong positive correlation between 100, 500, 2,000 and 6,000 m rowing speed and the muscle carnosine content in 18 elite Belgium rowers. Subjects were retested over 2,000 m after 7 weeks of supplementation with either 5 g·day^{-1} β-alanine or placebo, and showed a positive correlation between the increase in rowing speed and the increase in M-Carn. This would seem to have possible applications to rowing, and, kayak and canoe racing.

Conclusion

It remains to be established which areas of exercise are limited by pH decrease, but most certainly high-intensity exercising lasting ~1–6 min would likely benefit from an increase in M-Carn (table 1). It follows that the greater the increase in M-Carn then potentially the greater effect on exercise performance. Our current understanding is that competitive events with duration times of 1–6 min will be amongst those likely to gain. Table 1 provides some examples of Olympic events which fall into this time frame and might thus be positively affected by the use of β-alanine supplementation.

Disclosure Statement

R.C. Harris is named as an inventor on various patents owned by Natural Alternatives International, California, USA, relating to the use of supplemental β-alanine to increase muscle carnosine and exercise performance, the subject of this review. R.C. Harris retired from academic life in 2009 but continues to work as a consultant to Natural Alternatives International. T. Stellingwerff serves on a scientific advisory board for PowerBar/Nestlé Nutrition.

References

1 Abe H: Role of histidine-related compounds as intracellular proton buffering constituents in vertebrate muscle. Biochemistry (Mosc) 2000;65:757–765.

2 Harris RC, Wise JA, Price KA, et al: Determinants of muscle carnosine content. Amino Acids 2012;43:5–12.

3 Hill CA, Harris RC, Kim HJ, et al: Influence of beta-alanine supplementation on skeletal muscle carnosine concentrations and high intensity cycling capacity. Amino Acids 2007; 32:225–233.

4 Kendrick IP, Kim HJ, Harris RC, et al: The effect of 4 weeks beta-alanine supplementation and isokinetic training on carnosine concentrations in type I and II human skeletal muscle fibres. Eur J Appl Physiol 2009;106:131–138.

5 Stellingwerff T, Anwander H, Egger A, et al: Effect of two beta-alanine dosing protocols on muscle carnosine synthesis and washout. Amino Acids 2012;42:2461–2472.

6 Harris RC, Jones GA, Hill CA, et al: The carnosine content of V Lateralis in vegetarians and omnivores; in FASEB – Federation of American Societies for Experimental Biology, Washington, April 28 to May 2, 2007.

7 Everaert I, Mooyaart A, Baguet A, et al: Vegetarianism, female gender and increasing age, but not CNDP1 genotype, are associated with reduced muscle carnosine levels in humans. Amino Acids 2011;40:1221–1229.

8 Baguet A, Everaert I, Achten E, et al: The influence of sex, age and heritability on human skeletal muscle carnosine content. Amino Acids 2012;43:13–20.

9 Suzuki Y, Ito O, Takahashi H, Takamatsu K: The effect of sprint training on skeletal muscle carnosine in humans. Int J Sport Health Sci 2004;2:105–110.

10 Mannion AF, Jakeman PM, Willan PL: Effects of isokinetic training of the knee extensors on high-intensity exercise performance and skeletal muscle buffering. Eur J Appl Physiol Occup Physiol 1994;68:356–361.

11 Kendrick IP, Harris RC, Kim HJ, et al: The effects of 10 weeks of resistance training combined with beta-alanine supplementation on whole body strength, force production, muscular endurance and body composition. Amino Acids 2008;34:547–554.

12 Tallon MJ, Harris RC, Boobis LH, et al: The carnosine content of vastus lateralis is elevated in resistance-trained bodybuilders. J Strength Cond Res 2005;19:725–729.

13 Parkhouse WS, McKenzie DC, Hochachka PW, Ovalle WK: Buffering capacity of deproteinized human vastus lateralis muscle. J Appl Physiol 1985;58:14–17.

14 Hultman E, Sahlin K: Acid-base balance during exercise. Exerc Sport Sci Rev 1980;8:41–128.

15 Sahlin K, Harris RC: The creatine kinase reaction: a simple reaction with functional complexity. Amino Acids 2011;40:1363–1367.

16 Fabiato A, Fabiato F: Effects of pH on the myofilaments and the sarcoplasmic reticulum of skinned cells from cardiac and skeletal muscles. J Physiol 1978;276:233–255.

17 Dutka TL, Lamb GD: Effect of carnosine on excitation-contraction coupling in mechanically-skinned rat skeletal muscle. J Muscle Res Cell Motil 2004;25:203–213.

18 Dutka TL, Lamboley CR, McKenna MJ, et al: Effects of carnosine on contractile apparatus Ca^{2+} sensitivity and sarcoplasmic reticulum Ca^{2+} release in human skeletal muscle fibers. J Appl Physiol 2012;112:728–736.

19 Stellingwerff T, Decombaz J, Harris RC, Boesch C: Optimizing human in vivo dosing and delivery of beta-alanine supplements for muscle carnosine synthesis. Amino Acids 2012;43:57–65.

20 Harris RC, Tallon MJ, Dunnett M, et al: The absorption of orally supplied beta-alanine and its effect on muscle carnosine synthesis in human vastus lateralis. Amino Acids 2006;30:279–289.

21 Thwaites DT, Anderson CM: H+-coupled nutrient, micronutrient and drug transporters in the mammalian small intestine. Exp Physiol 2007;92:603–619.

22 Baguet A, Reyngoudt H, Pottier A, et al: Carnosine loading and washout in human skeletal muscles. J Appl Physiol 2009;106:837–842.

23 Decombaz J, Beaumont M, Vuichoud J, et al: Effect of slow-release beta-alanine tablets on absorption kinetics and paresthesia. Amino Acids 2012;43:67–76.

24 Crozier RA, Ajit SK, Kaftan EJ, Pausch MH: MrgD activation inhibits KCNQ/M-currents and contributes to enhanced neuronal excitability. J Neurosci 2007;27:4492–4496.

25 Sale C, Saunders B, Hudson S, et al: Effect of beta-alanine plus sodium bicarbonate on high-intensity cycling capacity. Med Sci Sports Exerc 2011;43:1972–1978.

26 del Favero S, Roschel H, Solis MY, et al: Beta-alanine (Carnosyn) supplementation in elderly subjects (60–80 years): effects on muscle carnosine content and physical capacity. Amino Acids 2012;43:49–56.

27 Saunders B, Sale C, Harris RC, Sunderland C: Effect of beta-alanine supplementation on repeated sprint performance during the Loughborough Intermittent Shuttle Test. Amino Acids 2012;43:39–47.

28 Saunders B, Sunderland C, Harris RC, Sale C: Beta-alanine supplementation improves YoYo intermittent recovery test performance. J Int Soc Sports Nutr 2012;9:39.

29 Hobson RM, Saunders B, Ball G, et al: Effects of beta-alanine supplementation on exercise performance: a meta-analysis. Amino Acids 2012;43:25–37.

30 Sale C, Saunders B, Harris RC: Effect of beta-alanine supplementation on muscle carnosine concentrations and exercise performance. Amino Acids 2010;39:321–333.

31 Baguet A, Bourgois J, Vanhee L, et al: Important role of muscle carnosine in rowing performance. J Appl Physiol 2010;109:1096–1101.

32 Sale C, Hill CA, Ponte J, Harris RC: Beta-alanine supplementation improves isometric endurance of the knee extensor muscles. J Int Soc Sports Nutr 2012;9:26.

33 Jagim AR, Wright GA, Brice AG, Doberstein ST: Effects of beta-alanine supplementation on sprint endurance. J Strength Cond Res 2013;27:526–532.

34 Van Thienen R, Van Proeyen K, Vanden Eynde B, et al: Beta-alanine improves sprint performance in endurance cycling. Med Sci Sports Exerc 2009;41:898–903.

35 Stout JR, Cramer JT, Zoeller RF, et al: Effects of beta-alanine supplementation on the onset of neuromuscular fatigue and ventilatory threshold in women. Amino Acids 2007;32:381–386.

36 Stout JR, Graves BS, Smith AE, et al: The effect of beta-alanine supplementation on neuromuscular fatigue in elderly (55–92 years): a double-blind randomized study. J Int Soc Sports Nutr 2008;5:21–26.

37 Baguet A, Koppo K, Pottier A, Derave W: Beta-alanine supplementation reduces acidosis but not oxygen uptake response during high-intensity cycling exercise. Eur J Appl Physiol 2010;108:495–503.

van Loon LJC, Meeusen R (eds): Limits of Human Endurance.
Nestlé Nutr Inst Workshop Ser, vol 76, pp 73–84, (DOI: 10.1159/000350259)
Nestec Ltd., Vevey/S. Karger AG., Basel, © 2013

Dietary Protein for Muscle Hypertrophy

Kevin D. Tipton[a] · Stuart M. Phillips[b]

[a]Health and Exercise Sciences Research Group, University of Stirling, Stirling, Scotland, UK;
[b]Department of Kinesiology, MacMaster University, Hamilton, ON, Canada

Abstract

Skeletal muscle hypertrophy is a beneficial adaptation for many individuals. The metabolic basis for muscle hypertrophy is the balance between the rates of muscle protein synthesis (MPS) and muscle protein breakdown (MPB), i.e. net muscle protein balance (NMPB = MPS − MPB). Resistance exercise potentiates the response of muscle to protein ingestion for up to 24 h following the exercise bout. Ingestion of many protein sources in temporal proximity (immediately before and at least within 24 h after) to resistance exercise increases MPS resulting in positive NMPB. Moreover, it seems that not all protein sources are equal in their capacity to stimulate MPS. Studies suggest that ~20–25 g of a high-quality protein maximizes the response of MPS following resistance exercise, at least in young, resistance-trained males. However, more protein may be required to maximize the response of MPS with less than optimal protein sources and/or with older individuals. Ingestion of carbohydrate with protein does not seem to increase the response of MPS following exercise. The response of inactive muscle to protein ingestion is impaired. Ingestion of a high-quality protein within close temporal proximity of exercise is recommended to maximize the potential for muscle growth.

Introduction

Skeletal muscle hypertrophy is a beneficial adaptation for many athletes, as well as other populations, including older adults, insulin resistant/diabetic individuals and others. Probably the most effective stimulus for muscle hypertrophy is resistance exercise. The hypertrophic response to resistance exercise is enhanced by nutrition, in particular provision of protein. Thus, study of the interaction of nutrition and exercise offers valuable information that may be used to enhance muscle hypertrophy and alter body composition during training.

Metabolic Basis for Muscle Hypertrophy

The metabolic basis for muscle hypertrophy is the balance between the rates of muscle protein synthesis (MPS) and muscle protein breakdown (MPB), i.e., net muscle protein balance (NMPB = MPS − MPB). The processes of MPS and MPB occur concurrently and either or both may change in response to the nutrition and exercise circumstances at a given time. NMPB alternates between positive and negative periods throughout the day depending on proximity to a protein-containing meal. Periods of positive NMPB must be of larger duration and magnitude than negative periods over any given time for muscle growth to occur. In particular, changes in the balance of the muscle myofibrillar proteins are responsible for changes in muscle mass since they comprise the majority of muscle proteins. Studies over the past 15 years or so indicate that it is predominantly changes in the rate of MPS in response to exercise and nutritional perturbations that have a much greater impact on changes in NMPB than changes in MPB [1–3].

Methodological Considerations

The importance of protein consumption for muscle hypertrophy may be investigated by both chronic longitudinal resistance training studies and acute metabolic studies examining MPS and in some cases MPB. Chronic studies assess changes in muscle mass and strength over a given time period, often from 6 up to 16 weeks, but rarely for longer periods. The acute metabolic studies assess the response of muscle anabolism, often in the form of MPS, to exercise plus some sort of nutrient ingestion. For the acute studies to be meaningful, an assumption is that the metabolic response to exercise and nutrition over a period of only a few hours represents the potential for an intervention to influence muscle growth over the longer term.

Intuitively, it is easier to accept that long-term training studies measuring changes in muscle mass are better to discern the influence of diet or dietary components on muscle hypertrophy. However, the control, expense and difficulty of performing these studies make them less than ideal. Longitudinal studies are often small, and physiologically important changes may not be detected due to limitations in measurement methods and/or variation in the response of individual participants. These difficulties may easily obscure the interpretation of results from these studies. Nevertheless, ultimately longitudinal end point studies can make important contributions to the body of knowledge concerning protein and muscle growth.

An alternative method to longitudinal studies for assessment of the efficacy of nutritional interventions to stimulate muscle hypertrophy is to perform acute metabolic studies. Over the past 15–20 years, stable isotopic tracer methodology has been used to investigate the response of MPS, MPB and NMPB to various nutrition and exercise combinations. The assumption is that the acute, i.e. over a few hours around the exercise, response to an intervention is representative of the muscle hypertrophy that would occur over a longer period of time. There is now evidence that this assumption is valid. Recently, several studies have demonstrated that the muscle hypertrophy over several weeks of resistance exercise training mirrors the acute response of MPS and NMPB [4, 5]. Thus, the acute metabolic response may be considered predictive of the potential for muscle hypertrophy. It should be noted that the predictive capacity of the acute studies is qualitative, rather than quantitative. Nevertheless, we propose that acute studies measuring MPS in response to resistance exercise and nutrition provide important information that may be used to design programs that will lead to muscle growth in various populations. Accordingly, this review will focus primarily on results from these acute metabolic studies.

Importance of Protein

Protein intake in conjunction with resistance exercise enhances the anabolic response of muscle. Elevated blood amino acid levels from infusion of amino acids or ingestion of a source of amino acids stimulates MPS resulting in positive NMPB [2, 6–8]. Moreover, it seems clear that it is the essential amino acids (EAAs) in the protein that are the key to muscle anabolism, i.e. provision of nonessential amino acids are unnecessary for stimulation of MPS [9]. However, it is unknown at this time whether someone could achieve an optimal MPS response and net balance consuming only EAAs. What we do know is that the response of muscle anabolism to exercise plus amino acids is greater than either alone [2]. Exercise potentiates the protein synthetic response in muscle allowing it to respond to provision of amino acids. Thus, the response of MPS, and specifically of the myofibrillar protein fraction, to protein ingestion is superior following exercise versus that seen at rest [10]. This response leads to muscle hypertrophy with repeated bouts of resistance exercise.

Recent work illustrates the importance of resistance exercise to potentiate the anabolic response of muscle to dietary protein. Witard et al. [11] demonstrated that MPS is elevated following exercise subsequent to a high protein meal consumed 3 h prior to the exercise. It is now clear that the amino acids from exogenous protein are being incorporated into the muscle protein following exercise.

Work from the laboratory of Prof. Luc van Loon using intrinsically labeled protein clearly demonstrates that incorporation of ingested amino acids, as well as endogenous amino acids, is increased by prior exercise [12]. Thus, the synergy of resistance exercise and ingested protein provide the optimal anabolic response of muscle that presumably leads to muscle growth.

Type of Protein

It is clear that ingestion of many protein sources in temporal proximity (immediately prior and at least within 24 h after) to resistance exercise increases MPS resulting in positive NMPB. Moreover, it seems that not all protein sources are equal in their capacity to stimulate MPS. Whereas studies have begun to elucidate the differences in the response of MPS during post-exercise recovery to various sources of protein, it is still difficult to unequivocally state that one source is ideal. Dairy proteins seem to offer some advantage for muscle anabolism over other protein sources. Wilkinson et al. [5] demonstrated that MPS was greater, resulting in greater positive NMPB with ingestion of fluid low fat milk compared to an isonitrogenous soy protein drink following resistance exercise. Moreover, when milk was ingested following each exercise bout during 12 weeks of resistance training, gains of muscle mass and strength were greater than when soy protein was ingested [4]. Subsequently, Tang et al. [7] demonstrated that the response of MPS to whey protein ingestion following resistance exercise was superior to that of either casein or soy protein. Similarly, myofibrillar MPS was greater with ingestion of whey protein isolate than micellar casein in older men following exercise [13] and at rest [13, 14]. These results suggest that dairy proteins – in particular whey protein – provide a superior anabolic response compared to other proteins.

The differences in the anabolic response to whey protein ingestion and the ingestion of other proteins likely is due to a combination of its high leucine and EAA content and the rapidity of digestion of the protein resulting in rapid hyperaminoacidemia. Data suggest that EAAs are the key to increasing MPS and NMPB with protein ingestion following resistance exercise [9]. In particular, the branched-chain amino acid leucine seems to be unique among the EAAs as a key regulator of translation initiation of MPS [3, 15]. Whey protein provides all of the EAAs, including leucine, in greater amounts than is present in human muscle protein, but soy and casein do not. In fact, recently, a 'leucine trigger' has been suggested to be a key factor for muscle anabolism. This thesis suggests that a threshold of leucine must be reached in the intramuscular pool before the maximal rate of MPS is stimulated. However, elevated leucine alone is insufficient to fully stimulate MPS [16]. Despite stimulation of translation initiation by leucine, provision of the other amino acids, e.g., from an intact protein source, is necessary to supply the substrate for MPS. Thus, the amino acid composition of whey protein seems to be an important component leading to superior responses of MPS following exercise.

Digestive properties of the various proteins likely contribute to differences in the response of MPS following exercise. Rapid appearance of amino acids into the blood seems to be important for an optimal response of MPS [17]. Since whey protein is digested more quickly than micellar casein, hyperaminoacidemia develops more rapidly. Greater and more rapid aminoacidemia of EAAs likely contributes to the superior anabolic response noted for whey protein over casein. Since micellar casein coagulates and precipitates when it is exposed to acid, the curd (a complex of fat, if present in the milk, and protein) that is formed is digested more slowly. Thus, a more moderate but prolonged hyperaminoacidemia results from casein ingestion [13]. Taken together, the data suggest that the superiority of whey protein for stimulation of MPS following exercise results from a rapid increase in amino acid, in particular leucine, availability. This sentiment would also be true about meals that, due to their mixed macronutrient composition, will have slower digestion kinetics and thus will lead to a slower and protracted aminoacidemia. So the digestive kinetics resemble those of casein more than they do whey. As such, at this point, all we can say is that intact isolated proteins, if they are digested rapidly and have a high leucine content, work well. However, we know nothing about mixed meal consumption and the effect of protein in a matrix of fat and carbohydrate.

The superiority of the anabolic response to whey protein is not a universal finding. Previously, similar NMPB was observed with ingestion of whey protein and casein following resistance exercise [18]. These results are seemingly at odds with other data suggesting that MPS was greater with greater whey protein ingestion [7, 13]. Whereas there was no difference in NMPB between whey and casein protein, a direct measurement of MPS was not made [18]. Thus, it is possible that MPS was greater with the whey protein, and MPB was less with casein ingestion resulting in similar NMPB [18]. On the other hand, the form of the ingested casein may be the key. Micellar casein is digested more slowly than whey protein resulting in a less rapid increase in aminoacidemia. Caseinate was used to stimulate muscle anabolism in the previous study [18]. This notion is supported by recent studies from Copenhagen. These studies reported no differences in the response of MPS to ingestion of whey protein and caseinate [19]. Thus, the form of protein may impact the pattern of aminoacidemia leading to differences in the anabolic response. Pennings et al. [14] also showed recently that hydrolysis of casein prior to ingestion resulted in a more rapid aminoacidemia and greater MPS response than micellar casein, but that whey was superior to both micellar and hydrolyzed casein.

Muscle Protein Breakdown

Most studies measure only MPS in response to protein ingestion and exercise or their combination. We fully acknowledge that MPB also is stimulated with resistance exercise in the fasted state [1, 20]. However, when protein is provided (infusion of amino acids or ingestion), the rise in post-exercise MPB is ablated. It has been argued that this amino acid-induced 'shutting off' of MPB is due to the increased intracellular amino acid availability preventing an increase in MPB that was needed to 'fuel' the increase in MPS [1]. It appears, however, that this idea may not be correct and instead that the rise in insulin that often accompanies hyperaminoacidemia may be responsible for reducing MPB [21]. This argument is not to dismiss the importance of measuring MPB, which is regulated by at least four different systems, but it is known that the feeding and exercise-induced fluctuation in MPS is 3–4 times that of MPB, so in healthy persons the role of MPB in determining muscle protein balance is much less relevant versus MPS.

Amount of Protein

It is well established that protein ingestion following exercise stimulates MPS. However, the optimal amount of protein has yet to be firmly established. Moore et al. [22] examined the response of mixed MPS to ingestion of varying amounts of egg protein following resistance exercise. MPS increased stepwise in response to 0, 5, 10 and 20 g of protein. However, the response to 40 g was not significantly greater than that of 20 g. Moreover, leucine oxidation increased dramatically with ingestion of 40 g of protein. Thus, it was determined that ~20 g of protein is sufficient to optimally stimulate MPS following exercise. Ingestion of more than 20 g simply results in oxidation of the excess amino acids [22]. Recently, we found that the response of myofibrillar MPS to whey protein was similar, i.e. the response to 40 g was not significantly greater than to 20 g [Witard et al., in prep.]. Moreover, the exercise was performed ~3 h following a meal, rather than in the fasted state. This amount (20 g) also maximized MPS in non-exercised muscle. As with the earlier results [22], amino acid oxidation and urea production were dramatically increased when 40 g of whey protein were ingested [Witard et al., in prep.]. Thus, it seems that ~20 g of a high-quality protein maximizes the response of MPS following resistance exercise, at least in young, resistance-trained males.

The response to varying doses of protein is influenced by factors other than simply the amount of protein. Similar to the results from young males [Witard et al., in prep.], Yang et al. [23] recently reported that 20 g of whey protein was sufficient to maximally stimulate myofibrillar MPS in non-exercised muscle. On the other hand, 40 g of whey protein was necessary to maximally stimulate myofibrillar MPS following exercise in older males [23]. Moreover, the type of protein impacts the dose response in older men. Soy protein ingestion (20 and 40 g) did not result in increased MPS in non-exercised muscle of older males [24]. However, with the anabolic potentiation of resistance exercise, myofibrillar MPS was increased by ingestion of 40 g, but not 20 g, of soy protein. When compared to whey protein, the response of MPS to soy protein was inferior. Thus, it seems that 40 g of protein is necessary for the optimal stimulation of MPS in older adults – a protein dose twice as great as that in young persons.

Timing of Protein Ingestion

It is clear that ingestion of protein in association with resistance exercise results in stimulation of MPS leading to positive NMPB and muscle growth; however, the precise timing of the ingestion in relation to the exercise may impact the response. Many feel that immediate (within as little as 45 min) post-exercise protein ingestion is crucial for the optimal response of muscle anabolism. This post-exercise period has been dubbed the 'window of anabolic potential', and whole books have been written supporting its importance. Clearly, early post-exercise ingestion of protein [7, 13, 17] or free amino acids [9, 25] results in increased MPS. Thus, immediate post-exercise ingestion of an amino acid source obviously is a sound method of enhancing muscle anabolism.

A training study from a Copenhagen laboratory may be the basis for the limited anabolic window purported by other authors. In that study, older men performed resistance exercise training for 12 weeks [26]. One group of volunteers consumed a protein-containing supplement immediately after exercise, whereas a second group waited 2 h to consume the supplement. Muscle mass in the group that waited 2 h to consume the protein did not increase, and the strength increase was much less than in the group that consumed protein immediately following exercise. Thus, it was concluded that waiting to consume protein not only inhibited, but also completely prevented, the anabolic response [26].

The notion that protein must be consumed immediately after exercise to have an anabolic impact is countered by data from studies on the acute anabolic response of muscle to feeding. MPS and NMPB were similar when EAA was ingested at 1 and 3 h following resistance exercise [27]. Moreover, the re-

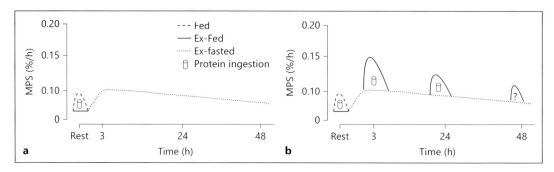

Fig. 1. Response of MPS to protein feeding at rest and resistance exercise in the fasted state (**a**) and protein feeding over 48 h after the exercise (**b**). Resistance exercise potentiates the muscle to respond to the anabolic stimulation of hyperaminoacidemia after protein ingestion for at least 24 h and up to 48 h after exercise. **a** From Phillips et al. [1]. **b** From Churchward-Venne et al. [3].

sponse was actually greater when those nutrients were ingested prior to exercise compared to immediately after exercise [25]. At the very least, these data suggest that the 'anabolic window' is slightly broader than the first hour or two after exercise. Nevertheless, these time points may still be considered within close proximity of exercise. Moreover, the form in which an amino acid source is ingested seems to influence the anabolic response to the timing of ingestion. Whereas EAA ingestion prior to exercise results in a superior anabolic response to ingestion following exercise [25], the response to ingestion of intact whey protein prior to and following exercise was shown to be similar [8]. As with other factors influencing the anabolic response, these differences likely are due to the digestive properties of the source of amino acids.

More recent work suggests that this 'window of opportunity' may be even more extensive than just a few hours around the exercise bout. The response of MPS to resistance exercise is greatest within the first few hours following the exercise bout, but the response lasts for up to 48 h [1]. Thus, it is logical to suggest that the influence of the exercise on the ability of the muscle to respond to hyperaminoacidemia would still be enhanced. In fact, Burd et al. [28] recently demonstrated that the synergistic response of muscle to exercise and nutrition lasts for at least 24 h. Whey protein ingestion 24 h following exercise resulted in superior rates of MPS compared to ingestion at rest [28]. These results suggest that the 'window of anabolic potential' lasts for at least 24 h, and possibly as long as 48 h, following exercise (fig. 1). Thus, whereas the optimal response may occur when protein is ingested soon after exercise, a normal post-exercise feeding pattern will, in fact, support muscle anabolism.

Coingestion of Other Nutrients with Protein

The bulk of research regarding the nutritional influences on muscle anabolism has focused on protein. However, both carbohydrates and fats are typically consumed with protein in a mixed meal. Thus, investigation of the impact of the other macronutrients may give some insight into optimization of muscle anabolism. There is very little information on the role of fat ingestion in the anabolic response of muscle following exercise. One study suggests that the fat content of milk may play a role in this response. The increase in NMPB following ingestion of whole milk was greater compared to that to ingestion of an isonitrogenous amount of fat-free milk [6]. The mechanism for this response is unknown, but blood flow may play a role. Thus, it seems that coingestion of fat with protein following exercise may warrant further investigation.

Whereas ingestion of fat with protein has not received much attention, ingestion of carbohydrate alone and with protein has been studied. The response of muscle protein metabolism to carbohydrate is thought to be due to the hyperinsulinemia. Earlier work demonstrated that hyperinsulinemia following resistance exercise contributed little to the response of MPS, but did impact NMPB due to a reduction in protein breakdown [29]. Subsequent work has confirmed that ingestion of carbohydrate with sufficient amounts of protein does not further increase MPS following exercise [30, 31]. Thus, both fat and carbohydrate may play a role in muscle anabolism following exercise.

Inactivity

It has been known for some time that inactivity reduces MPS [32] and that even a mild contractile stimulus like electrical stimulation can ablate this decline [33]. What we do know is that the reduction in fasted-state MPS also extends to the fed state at both low and high doses of amino acids [34]. Thus, inactivity and unloading induce a state of 'anabolic resistance' of the muscle to amino acids similar to that seen in the elderly [35]. It is unknown as to the cause of the inactivity-induced anabolic resistance, but it could be due to one or more of the following: reduced amino acid delivery as a result of an impaired insulin-mediated vasodilation [36], signaling defects inherent to the muscle itself, and/or another inactivity-related unknown mechanism. Whatever the mechanism, the fact remains that in a state of inactivity humans lose their ability to build protein. Interventions to prevent this decline from a nutrient standpoint have met with mixed success. Paddon-Jones [37] reported that consumption of a mixture of 16.5 g of EAAs (~35 g of high-quality protein) and 30 g of carbohydrate thrice daily preserved MPS, muscle strength, and skeletal muscle mass during 28 days of bed rest. The data from Paddon-Jones contrast somewhat with the findings of Trappe et al. [38] who reported no benefit of daily supplementation with a leucine-enriched whey protein supplement in women on 60 days of bed rest. In fact, the whey-supplemented group lost more leg muscle mass than the control (i.e. non-supplemented) group. Thus, it may be that in the short term (i.e. 4 weeks or less) amino acid supplementation is effective in attenuating muscle mass loss due to inactivity, but in the long term supplements are ineffective.

Conclusions and Recommendations

It is clear that the training impulse is the most important aspect of muscle hypertrophy. Nevertheless, it is equally certain that nutrition, particularly protein nutrition, may have an important influence. Current knowledge allows us to make a few recommendations to optimize the anabolic response to protein ingestion. First, it is clear that the total amount of protein consumed is not the most important factor to consider. Many other aspects of protein feeding play a role, including the amount, timing and source of protein, as well as coingestion of other nutrients with the protein. Thus, even consuming the same total amount of protein, utilization of these other factors could change the anabolic response. Consumption of ~20–25 g of high-quality, i.e. with ample leucine resulting in rapid hyperaminoacidemia, protein, e.g. whey protein, is sufficient to optimize the response, at least in healthy young males. Older individuals may need more protein for optimal muscle anabolism. Moreover, it is unclear if the total mass of muscle or the mass that is exercised will influence the response. Thus, a 50-kg gymnast may need less protein. The recommendation could perhaps be tailored to body mass. So, based on the body mass from earlier studies [22; Witard et al., in prep.], ~0.25–0.3 g protein/kg body mass could be recommended. Whereas, it is likely best to ingest protein soon after exercise, it seems clear that muscle does respond to protein ingestion for at least 24 h following exercise. Thus, all meals within that time will contribute to muscle hypertrophy. Ingestion of carbohydrate and perhaps even fat along with protein may contribute to muscle growth. Given the benefit of replenishing glycogen with carbohydrate ingestion, adding carbohydrate to protein is likely also prudent.

Disclosure Statement

The authors of this chapter have no financial arrangements to disclose.

References

1 Phillips SM, Tipton KD, Aarsland A, et al: Mixed muscle protein synthesis and breakdown after resistance exercise in humans. Am J Physiol 1997;273:E99–E107.

2 Biolo G, Tipton KD, Klein S, Wolfe RR: An abundant supply of amino acids enhances the metabolic effect of exercise on muscle protein. Am J Physiol 1997;273:E122–E129.

3 Churchward-Venne TA, Burd NA, Phillips SM, Research Group EM: Nutritional regulation of muscle protein synthesis with resistance exercise: strategies to enhance anabolism. Nutr Metab (Lond) 2012;9:40.

4 Hartman JW, Tang JE, Wilkinson SB, et al: Consumption of fat-free fluid milk after resistance exercise promotes greater lean mass accretion than does consumption of soy or carbohydrate in young, novice, male weightlifters. Am J Clin Nutr 2007;86:373–381.

5 Wilkinson SB, Tarnopolsky MA, Macdonald MJ, et al: Consumption of fluid skim milk promotes greater muscle protein accretion after resistance exercise than does consumption of an isonitrogenous and isoenergetic soy-protein beverage. Am J Clin Nutr 2007; 85:1031–1040.

6 Elliot TA, Cree MG, Sanford AP, et al: Milk ingestion stimulates net muscle protein synthesis following resistance exercise. Med Sci Sports Exerc 2006;38:667–674.

7 Tang JE, Moore DR, Kujbida GW, et al: Ingestion of whey hydrolysate, casein, or soy protein isolate: effects on mixed muscle protein synthesis at rest and following resistance exercise in young men. J Appl Physiol 2009; 107:987–992.

8 Tipton KD, Elliott TA, Cree MG, et al: Stimulation of net muscle protein synthesis by whey protein ingestion before and after exercise. Am J Physiol Endocrinol Metab 2007; 292:E71–E76.

9 Tipton KD, Ferrando AA, Phillips SM, et al: Postexercise net protein synthesis in human muscle from orally administered amino acids. Am J Physiol 1999;276:E628–E634.

10 Moore DR, Tang JE, Burd NA, et al: Differential stimulation of myofibrillar and sarcoplasmic protein synthesis with protein ingestion at rest and after resistance exercise. J Physiol 2009;587:897–904.

11 Witard OC, Tieland M, Beelen M, et al: Resistance exercise increases postprandial muscle protein synthesis in humans. Med Sci Sports Exerc 2009;41:144–154.

12 Pennings B, Koopman R, Beelen M, et al: Exercising before protein intake allows for greater use of dietary protein-derived amino acids for de novo muscle protein synthesis in both young and elderly men. Am J Clin Nutr 2011;93:322–331.

13 Burd NA, Yang Y, Moore DR, et al: Greater stimulation of myofibrillar protein synthesis with ingestion of whey protein isolate v. Micellar casein at rest and after resistance exercise in elderly men. Br J Nutr 2012;108:958–962. DOI 10.1017/S0007114511006271.

14 Pennings B, Boirie Y, Senden JM, et al: Whey protein stimulates postprandial muscle protein accretion more effectively than do casein and casein hydrolysate in older men. Am J Clin Nutr 2011;93:997–1005.

15 Anthony JC, Anthony TG, Layman DK: Leucine supplementation enhances skeletal muscle recovery in rats following exercise. J Nutr 1999;129:1102–1106.

16 Churchward-Venne TA, Burd NA, Mitchell CJ, et al: Supplementation of a suboptimal protein dose with leucine or essential amino acids: effects on myofibrillar protein synthesis at rest and following resistance exercise in men. J Physiol 2012;590:2751–2765.

17 West DW, Burd NA, Coffey VG, et al: Rapid aminoacidemia enhances myofibrillar protein synthesis and anabolic intramuscular signaling responses after resistance exercise. Am J Clin Nutr 2011;94:795–803.

18 Tipton KD, Elliott TA, Cree MG, et al: Ingestion of casein and whey proteins result in muscle anabolism after resistance exercise. Med Sci Sports Exerc 2004;36:2073–2081.

19 Reitelseder S, Agergaard J, Doessing S, et al: Whey and casein labeled with l-[1-13c]leucine and muscle protein synthesis: effect of resistance exercise and protein ingestion. Am J Physiol Endocrinol Metab 2011;300:E231–E242.

20 Biolo G, Maggi SP, Williams BD, et al: Increased rates of muscle protein turnover and amino acid transport after resistance exercise in humans. Am J Physiol 1995;268:E514–E520.

21 Borsheim E, Cree MG, Tipton KD, et al: Effect of carbohydrate intake on net muscle protein synthesis during recovery from resistance exercise. J Appl Physiol 2004;96:674–678.

22 Moore DR, Robinson MJ, Fry JL, et al: Ingested protein dose response of muscle and albumin protein synthesis after resistance exercise in young men. Am J Clin Nutr 2008;89:161–168.

23 Yang Y, Breen L, Burd NA, et al: Resistance exercise enhances myofibrillar protein synthesis with graded intakes of whey protein in older men. Br J Nutr 2012;108:1780–1788.

24 Yang Y, Churchward-Venne TA, Burd NA, et al: Myofibrillar protein synthesis following ingestion of soy protein isolate at rest and after resistance exercise in elderly men. Nutr Metab (Lond) 2012;9:57.

25 Tipton KD, Rasmussen BB, Miller SL, et al: Timing of amino acid-carbohydrate ingestion alters anabolic response of muscle to resistance exercise. Am J Physiol Endocrinol Metab 2001;281:E197–E206.

26 Esmarck B, Andersen JL, Olsen S, et al: Timing of postexercise protein intake is important for muscle hypertrophy with resistance training in elderly humans. J Physiol 2001;535:301–311.

27 Rasmussen BB, Tipton KD, Miller SL, et al: An oral essential amino acid-carbohydrate supplement enhances muscle protein anabolism after resistance exercise. J Appl Physiol 2000;88:386–392.

28 Burd NA, West DW, Moore DR, et al: Enhanced amino acid sensitivity of myofibrillar protein synthesis persists for up to 24 h after resistance exercise in young men. J Nutr 2011;141:568–573.

29 Biolo G, Williams BD, Fleming RY, Wolfe RR: Insulin action on muscle protein kinetics and amino acid transport during recovery after resistance exercise. Diabetes 1999;48:949–957.

30 Koopman R, Beelen M, Stellingwerff T, et al: Coingestion of carbohydrate with protein does not further augment postexercise muscle protein synthesis. Am J Physiol Endocrinol Metab 2007;293:E833–E842.

31 Staples AW, Burd NA, West DW, et al: Carbohydrate does not augment exercise-induced protein accretion versus protein alone. Med Sci Sports Exerc 2011;43:1154–1161.

32 Gibson JN, Halliday D, Morrison WL, et al: Decrease in human quadriceps muscle protein turnover consequent upon leg immobilization. Clin Sci (Lond) 1987;72:503–509.

33 Gibson JN, McMaster MJ, Scrimgeour CM, et al: Rates of muscle protein synthesis in paraspinal muscles: lateral disparity in children with idiopathic scoliosis. Clin Sci (Lond) 1988;75:79–83.

34 Glover EI, Phillips SM, Oates BR, et al: Immobilization induces anabolic resistance in human myofibrillar protein synthesis with low and high dose amino acid infusion. J Physiol 2008;586:6049–6061.

35 Cuthbertson D, Smith K, Babraj J, et al: Anabolic signaling deficits underlie amino acid resistance of wasting, aging muscle. FASEB J 2005;19:422–424.

36 Timmerman KL, Lee JL, Fujita S, et al: Pharmacological vasodilation improves insulin-stimulated muscle protein anabolism but not glucose utilization in older adults. Diabetes 2010;59:2764–2771.

37 Paddon-Jones D: Essential amino acid and carbohydrate supplementation ameliorates muscle protein loss in humans during 28 days bedrest. J Clin Endocrinol Metab 2004;89:4351–4358.

38 Trappe TA, Burd NA, Louis ES, et al: Influence of concurrent exercise or nutrition countermeasures on thigh and calf muscle size and function during 60 days of bed rest in women. Acta Physiol (Oxf) 2007;191:147–159.

van Loon LJC, Meeusen R (eds): Limits of Human Endurance.
Nestlé Nutr Inst Workshop Ser, vol 76, pp 85–102, (DOI: 10.1159/000350261)
Nestec Ltd., Vevey/S. Karger AG., Basel, © 2013

The Role of Amino Acids in Skeletal Muscle Adaptation to Exercise

Nick Aguirre[a] · Luc J.C. van Loon[b] · Keith Baar[a]

[a]University of California Davis, Davis, CA, USA; [b]Department of Human Movement Sciences, NUTRIM School for Nutrition, Toxicology and Metabolism, Maastricht University Medical Centre+, Maastricht, The Netherlands

Abstract

The synthesis of new protein is necessary for both strength and endurance adaptations. While the proteins that are made might differ, myofibrillar proteins following resistance exercise and mitochondrial proteins and metabolic enzymes following endurance exercise, the basic premise of shifting to a positive protein balance after training is thought to be the same. What is less clear is the contribution of nutrition to the adaptive process. Following resistance exercise, proteins rich in the amino acid leucine increase the activation of mTOR, the rate of muscle protein synthesis (MPS), and the rate of muscle mass and strength gains. However, an effect of protein consumption during acute post-exercise recovery on mitochondrial protein synthesis has yet to be demonstrated. Protein ingestion following endurance exercise does facilitate an increase in skeletal MPS, supporting muscle repair, growth and remodeling. However, whether this results in improved performance has yet to be demonstrated. The current literature suggests that a strength athlete will experience an increased sensitivity to protein feeding for at least 24 h after exercise, but immediate consumption of 0.25 g/kg bodyweight of rapidly absorbed protein will enhance MPS rates and drive the skeletal muscle hypertrophic response. At rest, ~0.25 g/kg bodyweight of dietary protein should be consumed every 4–5 h and another 0.25–0.5 g/kg bodyweight prior to sleep to facilitate the postprandial muscle protein synthetic response. In this way, consuming dietary protein can complement intense exercise training and facilitate the skeletal muscle adaptive response.   Copyright © 2013 Nestec Ltd., Vevey/S. Karger AG, Basel

Introduction

Muscular adaptation to resistance (muscle hypertrophy) and endurance (mitochondrial biogenesis and angiogenesis) type exercise is dependent on the de novo synthesis of myofibrillar and mitochondrial proteins, respectively [1]. The phenotype of bigger muscles in the strength athlete is the result of the rate of myofibrillar protein synthesis exceeding the rate of myofibrillar protein breakdown, whereas the endurance phenotype of more mitochondrial proteins occurs when this subset of proteins is synthesized faster than they are broken down. Therefore, protein balance (the sum of protein synthesis and breakdown) is key to determining the phenotypic adaptation to exercise training. Even though the rate of muscle protein breakdown increases following an acute bout of exercise [2], the corresponding increase in muscle protein synthesis (MPS) is 3- to 5-fold greater [2, 3]. Together with the methodological difficulties in measuring protein breakdown, this means that most research has focused on the regulation of protein synthesis after exercise.

In the fasted state, protein balance is negative. Resistance type exercise in the fasted state results in an increase in both protein synthesis and degradation [3]. Since the increase in synthesis is greater than the increase in degradation, net balance becomes less negative. However, in order for protein balance to become positive, an individual needs to consume a source of amino acids [4]. Tipton et al. [4] showed that when subjects consumed 40 g of either a mixed amino acid solution (containing both essential, EAAs, and non-essential amino acids) or an EAA solution (also containing arginine), MPS increased equally between supplemented groups and to a greater degree than in the fasted state, resulting in a positive protein balance. Therefore, resistance type exercise combined with provision of sufficient EAAs can shift net protein balance to positive. The effects of protein supplementation on mitochondrial protein synthesis have not been studied extensively. However, the early reports suggest that amino acid supplementation does not affect mitochondrial protein synthesis during the acute stages of post-exercise recovery [5]. This chapter will explore the mechanisms underlying the effects of amino acids on skeletal muscle adaptations and provides some practical suggestions based on these mechanisms in an effort to maximize the effects of training.

Adaptations to Strength Exercise

Resistance exercise, forcing a muscle to work close to or above its maximal isometric force to failure, results in an acute increase in MPS that can last more than 24 h [6, 7]. When repeated at a sufficient frequency, this transient increase in protein synthesis leads to an increase in muscle mass and strength. A number of cellular and molecular processes have been identified that transduce mechanical load into an increase in protein synthesis. Chief among these is the activation of the mTOR. In every model studied to date, loading results in the activation of mTOR, and the acute activation of mTOR is predictive of the gain in muscle mass and strength following more prolonged exercise training [8, 9]. Further, inhibiting mTOR with the macrolide antibiotic rapamycin blocks the acute increase in protein synthesis in people [10] and the increase in muscle mass in rodents [11, 12], suggesting that mTOR activation is required for muscle hypertrophy. Interestingly, mTOR is initially activated by both resistance and endurance type exercise. However, only after resistance exercise is the activation of mTOR maintained for longer periods [1]. In fact, following resistance type exercise, mTOR can remain active for upwards of 18 h [13], suggesting that mTOR might drive the protein synthesis response to resistance type exercise.

mTOR

mTOR is a serine/threonine protein kinase with structural similarities to PI-3 kinase (phosphatidylinositol-3 kinase). On its own, mTOR has no catalytic activity. In order for mTOR to become a functional kinase, it has to form a complex with other proteins that stabilize its structure, move it to specific regions of the cell, and regulate its binding to target proteins [14]. There are two known complexes of mTOR (complex 1 and 2). Both of the complexes contain the G-protein β-subunit-like protein (GβL; also known as lsT8) and the DEP domain-containing mTOR-interacting protein (DEPTOR) [15] that positively and negatively regulate mTOR, respectively. mTORC2 is targeted to membranes through its interaction with mammalian stress-activated map kinase-interacting protein 1 (mSIN1) [16], and is held together by protein observed with rictor (PROTOR) 1 or 2 [17]. The two mTOR complexes phosphorylate different proteins due to the presence of either the regulatory-associated protein of mTOR (raptor) or rapamycin-insensitive companion of mTOR (rictor) [18]. In mTORC1, raptor binds to proteins that contain a TOS (TOR signaling) motif such as eukaryotic initiation factor (eIF) 4E binding protein-1 (4E-BP1) [19], the 70-kDa ribosomal protein S6 kinase (S6K1) [20], hypoxia-inducible factor-1 (HIF-1) [21], and proline-rich Akt substrate of 40 kDa (PRAS40) [22, 23]. In contrast, rictor directs mTOR towards akt/PKB (protein kinase B), serum- and glucocorticoid-induced protein kinase (SGK), and protein kinase C (PKC) [24].

The most studied targets of mTOR are 4E-BP1 and S6K1. Phosphorylation of 4E-BP1 by mTOR changes its shape and prevents it from binding to eIF4E [25]. Free eIF4E can then bind to two other initiation factors, eIF4G and eIF4A, to form eIF4F and promote translation initiation. When S6K1 is activated by mTOR, it phosphorylates and turns on eIF4B [26] and phosphorylates and turns off eukaryotic elongation factor 2 kinase (eEF2K) [27]. Activation of eIF4B increases the unwinding of secondary structure in mRNA so that they can be translated. This specifically increases the rate of translation of genes that are important in cell growth, such as fibroblast growth factor (bFGF) [28]. Inactivation of eEF2K prevents the phosphorylation of elongation factor 2 (eEF2), accelerating the elongation step and promoting protein synthesis. In this way, S6K1 contributes to the regulation of both translation initiation and elongation. Even though these are the most studied targets of mTOR, there is developing evidence that other targets of mTOR are more important for muscle hypertrophy [MacKenzie et al. unpubl. obs.]. To that end, the recent discovery of two novel kinases downstream of mTOR that lead to ribosome biogenesis and an increase in the capacity for protein synthesis is extremely exciting [29].

Activation of mTOR

mTOR activity is regulated by growth factors, nutrients, stress, and mechanical loading [30]. Of particular importance to this review is the role of amino acids in regulating the activation of mTOR. Amino acids can directly stimulate mTOR activity in the absence of changes in metabolic stress, growth factors, or mechanical loading. Amino acids mediate this effect by uniting mTOR and its activator Rheb (ras homologue enriched in brain) within the cell. Over the last few years, the mechanism underlying this complex process has been elucidated, and a number of novel molecular actors have been identified including: the vacuolar protein sorting-34 [31], the leucyl tRNA synthase (LRS) [32], Rag proteins [33], and the ragulator [34]. Vps34 is one of the oldest kinases in our genome [31] and functions primarily to move vesicles around within the cell. Since the mTOR activator Rheb is located on the membrane of a vesicle, activating Vps34 moves Rheb and increases the likelihood of interacting with mTOR. LRS is the enzyme that ligates the amino acid leucine onto tRNAs containing the sequence TTA, TTG, CTT, CTC, CTA, or CTG and therefore is required for the synthesis of proteins containing the amino acid leucine. The Rag proteins are a family of four small G proteins that form heterodimers and control the location of mTOR within the cell. The ragulator is a trimer of MP1, p14, and p18 that binds to active Rag heterodimers and brings mTOR to its activator Rheb. As illustrated in figure 1, when leucine enters it binds to and activates the LRS. Han et al. [32] elegantly showed that the LRS serves as a GTPase activating protein (GAP) towards RagD. When RagD is bound to GTP, the Rag complex is inactive. When LRS acts as a GAP towards RagD, RagD hydrolyzes its GTP to GDP.

After RagD hydrolyzes its GTP, the ragulator makes RagB release its GDP and bind GTP and in so doing activates the Rag complex. Once active, the Rag

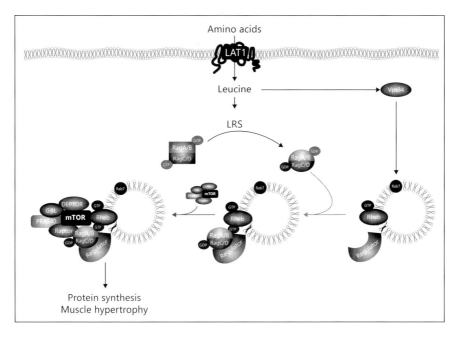

Amino acids

LAT1

Leucine

Vps34

LRS

RagA/B
RagC/D

RagA/B
RagC/D

Rab7

mTOR

Rab7

DEPTOR

GβL

mTOR   Rheb

PRAS40

Raptor   RagA/B

RagC/D

Regulator

Rheb

RagA/B
RagC/D

Regulator

Rheb

Regulator

Protein synthesis
Muscle hypertrophy

Fig. 1. Depiction of the activation of mTOR by amino acids. Leucine enters the muscle via LAT1, and through the LRS this activates the Rag complex. Through binding to raptor and the regulator, the Rag complex brings mTOR to its activator Rheb resulting in the activation of protein synthesis.

complex can bind to both raptor and the ragulator. Since the ragulator is located on the same vesicle as Rheb (the activator of mTOR), the net effect of leucine is to bring mTOR to its activator. If Rheb has been activated by either growth factors or mechanical loading, the result is an increase in mTOR activity and MPS. Interestingly, the other Rag heterodimer is not activated by the LRS [32], suggesting that there may be other amino acids or amino acid analogues that activate the RagA/RagC complex and by extension mTOR.

The Role of Leucine Uptake in Control of mTOR

As described above, leucine uptake is critical for activating mTOR via RagB/RagD and consequently increasing MPS. Following resistance type exercise in humans [3] and rats [13], the free leucine content of muscle is transiently increased, suggesting that the prolonged activation of mTOR could be mediated by a rise in intracellular leucine. From these data, it stands to logic that leucine entry into muscle could limit mTOR activation and the synergistic effect of resistance exercise and amino acid supplementation. The primary leucine transporter in muscle is the L-type amino acid transporter 1 (LAT1/SLC7A5). LAT1 transports leucine (along with other EAAs) into muscle in exchange for glutamine [35]. Glutamine and the other neutral amino acids are transported into muscle through the system A amino acid transporters: sodium-coupled neutral amino acid transporter 1 and 2 (SNAT2/SLC1A5) [36]. These transporters work in unison in what has been termed tertiary active transport. Primary active transport, where movement of ions is directly coupled with ATP consumption, of sodium through the Na^+/K^+-ATPase sets up the low intramuscular sodium gradient used for secondary active transport of glutamine through SNAT2. The glutamine gradient generated by SNAT2 in turn drives leucine influx and glutamine efflux through LAT1. Experimentally, this is observed as an increase in LAT1 transport of leucine when SNAT2 is coexpressed or an increase in leucine uptake when cells are pre-loaded with glutamine [35]. In contrast, mTOR signaling and protein synthesis are simultaneously decreased when leucine uptake is reduced due to SNAT2 inhibition [37, 38]. The data suggest that LAT1 and SNAT2 are important for mTOR activation.

With the importance of LAT1 and SNAT2 in leucine uptake and the transient increase in intramuscular leucine after resistance exercise, it is not surprising that LAT1 protein increases in skeletal muscle of young individuals following resistance exercise. Interestingly, Drummond et al. [39] found LAT1 protein and mTOR activity (S6 phosphorylation) increased significantly 6 and 24 h after resistance exercise in younger subjects, whereas in older subjects LAT1 protein did not increase and the activity of mTOR returned to baseline by 6 h. These data suggest that an increase in LAT1 protein is required for the prolonged activation of mTOR following loading, and the inability to increase LAT1 could underlie the anabolic resistance seen in old individuals. In agreement with this hypothesis, we have found that mice lacking LAT1 in their muscles show a marked reduction in mTOR activity 3 h after resistance exercise compared with wild-type mice [Aguirre and Baar, unpubl.]. Like resistance exercise, LAT1 and SNAT2 mRNA and protein increase after consuming EAA, and this increase occurs concomitant with mTOR activation [40]. Together, these data suggest that the activation of mTOR and the increase in protein synthesis after resistance exercise or amino acid feeding is dependent on leucine uptake through LAT1.

Resistance exercise, when combined with EAAs (specifically leucine), results in the prolonged activation of mTOR. In the absence of LAT1, this increase in mTOR activity is largely lost, suggesting that the uptake of leucine is an important trigger for mTOR activation and protein synthesis. This so-called 'leucine trigger' through LAT1 and the LRS not only forms the molecular mechanism underlying the activation of mTOR and protein synthesis, but also the practical consideration of which protein sources are more effective in facilitating the adaptive response in skeletal muscle in response to exercise training.

Protein Supplementation and Endurance Adaptations

The role of protein supplementation in the adaptation to endurance type exercise (i.e. the increase in mitochondrial protein synthesis) is far less studied than for resistance type exercise. From the limited studies performed to date, it does not appear that protein supplementation increases mitochondrial protein synthesis during the acute stages of post-exercise recovery. Specifically, Breen et al. [5] showed that adding 10 g of whey protein to a drink containing 25 g of carbohydrate had no effect on mitochondrial protein synthesis rates. With either drink, mitochondrial protein synthesis was increased from previously reported control levels [1]. However, the presence of whey protein after endurance type exercise did not affect mitochondrial protein synthesis rates, even though myofibrillar protein synthesis rates increased by ~50%. It could be speculated that the inability of protein ingestion following endurance type exercise to stimulate mitochondrial protein synthesis rates is due to mTOR not regulating mitochondrial protein synthesis [41]. In fact, in cell culture, treatment with the mTOR-specific inhibitor rapamycin actually increases cytochrome oxidase (COX) activity, COX IV protein, and mitochondrial transcription factor A levels [41]. This suggests that mTOR is not necessary to increase mitochondrial proteins, and therefore amino acid supplementation would not have a direct effect on muscle mitochondrial protein synthesis. However, it is possible that the time line of post-exercise stimulation of protein synthesis rates differs substantially for mitochondrial and myofibrillar proteins, making a direct comparison challenging. Since providing exogenous amino acids modulates skeletal MPS both by activating signaling pathways and by providing substrate for de novo MPS, it will be of key importance to identify the factors(s) that limit myofibrillar as well as mitochondrial MPS rates in vivo during acute and more prolonged post-exercise recovery.

Amino Acids Attenuate the Immunosuppression Response after Intense Exercise

The absence of a protein-dependent increase in mitochondrial protein synthesis does not mean that protein supplementation would not be beneficial for endurance performance. Besides the capacity of exogenous amino acids to modu-

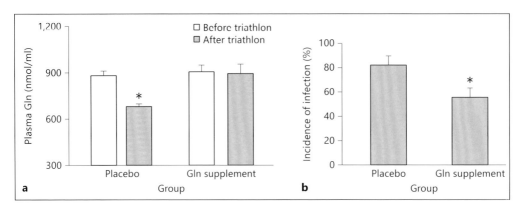

Fig. 2. Effect of glutamine (Gln) supplementation on plasma Gln (**a**) and incidence of infection (**b**) following an Olympic distance triathlon. Adapted from Castell and Newsholme [43] and Bassit et al. [46].

late post-exercise muscle protein synthetic and/or proteolytic signaling and provide precursors for MPS, there have been suggestions that amino acids may also be relevant for maintaining proper immune status during intense endurance type exercise training. Immediately following strenuous exercise, there is a transient suppression of the immune system that may lead to an 'open window' for infection [42]. This 'window' is proposed to last anywhere from 6 h to a week following exhaustive exercise, is directly related to the intensity and duration of exercise [43, 44], and can be exacerbated in an overtrained state [45]. One potential cause of this 'open window' may be a decline in glutamine bioavailability of more than 20% [43, 44, 46–49] likely due to accelerated glutamine metabolism by leukocytes [47–49]. Since glutamine is a metabolic substrate for many immune cells, including lymphocytes, macrophages and neutrophils, many experts hypothesize that the reduction in plasma glutamine and branched-chain amino acids (BCAA) after intense exercise promotes immunosuppression [42, 47–49]. Current evidence supports this hypothesis by linking lower plasma glutamine concentrations in middle-distance runners, marathoners, ultra-marathoners and elite rowers with impaired immune responses [43, 44, 46] and higher incidences of infection up to 7 days after intense training/competition (fig. 2) [43]. In these same experiments, supplementation with glutamine [43, 44] or BCAA [46] was effective at restoring circulating plasma glutamine to pre-exercise levels, as well as preventing immunosuppression and reducing athletes' reported infections [43]. BCAA having the same effect as glutamine on immunosuppression is likely due to the conversion of BCAA into glutamate [50] and enhanced export of glutamine into the bloodstream in the presence of BCAA [35].

The mechanism by which glutamine opposes immunosuppression is not completely understood, but recent findings suggest that glutamine consumed in conjunction with whey protein isolate improves lymphocyte function [51]. As discussed above, glutamine exchange with leucine through LAT1 is important in the activation of mTOR. Consistent with a role of mTOR in lymphocyte function, Sinclair et al. [52] have shown that rapamycin can redirect activated T cells to secondary organs such as the spleen and lymph nodes resulting in premature termination of immune responses. Ingestion of sufficient glutamine and leucine is likely required to increase leucine uptake and mTOR activation in the lymphocytes, through SNAT2 and LAT1, and as such to maintain proper immune function. Glutamine supplementation also decreases neutrophil apoptosis after a bout of endurance type exercise in part by enhancing antiapoptotic gene expression of bcl-xL and inhibits proapoptotic genes such as bax, bal, p53 and caspase 3 [53, 54]. These data suggest that ingestion of ample glutamine and BCAA may be beneficial for limiting the 'open window' for infection following intense exercise or competition. However, several recent glutamine feeding intervention studies indicate that although the plasma glutamine concentration can be kept constant during and after prolonged strenuous exercise, specific glutamine supplementation does not seem to prevent post-exercise changes in various aspects of immune function [55]. Although glutamine is essential for lymphocyte proliferation, the plasma glutamine concentration does not seem to fall sufficiently low after exercise to compromise the rate of proliferation [55]. Therefore, whether glutamine/BCAA supplementation will improve immune function in endurance athletes has yet to be determined conclusively.

Practical Considerations regarding Protein Supplementation

For sedentary adults, the Institute of Medicine recommends consumption of 0.8 $g \cdot kg^{-1} \cdot day^{-1}$ protein [56]. However, this recommendation is based on nitrogen balance studies and is unlikely to support proper adaptation to intense exercise training in athletes. The American College of Sports Medicine's (ACSM) position stand recommended protein intake ranges from 1.2 to 1.7 $g \cdot kg^{-1} \cdot day^{-1}$ for athletes [57]. In strength athletes, consuming protein near Institute of Medicine levels (0.86 $g \cdot kg^{-1} \cdot day^{-1}$) resulted in lower whole-body protein synthesis rates than a diet containing either 1.4 $g \cdot kg^{-1} \cdot day^{-1}$ or 2.4 $g \cdot kg^{-1} \cdot day^{-1}$ [58]. Interestingly, increasing dietary protein from 1.4 to 2.4 $g \cdot kg^{-1} \cdot day^{-1}$ did not further increase whole-body protein synthesis rates but stimulated amino acid oxidation. In endurance-trained athletes, 1.4 $g \cdot kg^{-1} \cdot day^{-1}$ has been recommended on the basis of nitrogen balance [59]. Overall, there does not seem to be any

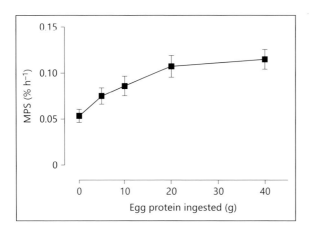

Fig. 3. Dose-response of MPS in relation to the amount of egg protein consumed after resistance exercise. Adapted from Moore et al. [61].

advantage for athletes when consuming more than the upper boundary of recommended protein intake described in the ACSM position even during intense training cycles [57]. In addition, it should be noted that overall dietary protein intake in most athletes is generally well above requirements as the greater energy intake with a diet containing more than 15% energy derived from protein translates in a daily protein intake well in excess over 1.4 g protein/kg per day. However, this does not imply that dietary protein supplementation cannot be of benefit to optimize skeletal muscle adaptation to exercise training as provision of the proper type and amount of dietary protein with the right timing can be of great importance when trying to optimize muscle reconditioning following exercise training and competition.

Protein Amount and the Adaptation to Exercise

Dose-response analysis of the rate of protein synthesis either at rest [60] or following resistance type exercise [61] has demonstrated that ingestion of 8–10 g of EAAs, roughly 20–25 g of a high-quality protein, maximizes mixed MPS rates in healthy young volunteers. At rest, ingestion of 10 g of EAA has been shown to result in peak postprandial MPS rates in healthy young males [60]. Following resistance exercise, there is an increase in amino acid sensitivity that increases the muscle protein synthetic response to protein and/or amino acid provision [62]. Consuming 20 g of whole egg protein, approximately 8 g of EAA, after resistance type exercise maximizes MPS rates (fig. 3) [61]. Increasing the amount of protein consumed, up to 40 g, resulted in only a marginal increase in mixed

MPS (11%), whereas protein oxidation increased significantly [61]. These data suggest that post-exercise ingestion of more than 20–25 g dietary protein will not be of much benefit. However, the latter may be restricted to young adults as larger amounts of dietary protein need to be ingested to maximize postprandial MPS in older individuals [63, 64], indicating that our sensitivity to amino acids may decline with aging [39, 40].

Protein Timing and the Adaptation to Exercise

The dose-response experiments suggest that ingestion of 20–25 g of a high-quality protein will maximize mixed MPS rates. Consequently, this amount of protein should be consumed at various intervals throughout the day. However, the length of the intervals between protein meals remains to be fully determined. We know that prolonged exposure to elevated amino acid concentrations can induce insulin resistance through a feedback mechanism initiated by mTOR [65]. In fact, chronic elevation of plasma amino acids levels does not maintain elevated MPS rates [66], and is therefore unlikely to benefit skeletal muscle adaptation. In support of this concept, Moore et al. [67] demonstrated that after ingesting 25 g whey protein following myofibrillar protein synthesis returned to baseline levels after 5 h of postprandial recovery. Therefore, to optimize postprandial MPS, it is advised to provide 20–25 g dietary protein every 4–5 h.

Recent work suggests that it might also be of benefit to provide some protein prior to an overnight fast. Preventing muscle protein balance from becoming negative during sleep may facilitate the muscle protein synthetic response to exercise and improve muscle reconditioning. 40 g of casein consumed 30 min before going to sleep was shown to be properly digested and absorbed throughout the night, and more importantly this amount of protein strongly stimulated (~22%) MPS [68, 69]. Together, these data suggest that athletes who are looking to increase lean mass should be consuming ~25 g of protein every 4–5 h throughout the day and a further 25–40 g of protein prior to sleep.

For many athletes though, increasing lean body mass is not the goal. The goal for these athletes is to improve protein turnover in muscles that are important for performance but without overall changes in bodyweight. For these individuals, a more restrictive diet together with timed protein intake will be more effective. Rather than consuming protein throughout the day, these individuals should be advised to consume fewer calories throughout the day and then supplement their diet with protein in conjunction with their workouts. Taking a little protein or amino acids prior to and/or during resistance type exercise results in greater post-exercise MPS than taking the same supplement after the exercise bout. This is likely attributed to a more rapid provision of dietary protein-derived amino acids that will be available directly after cessation of exercise [70]. Furthermore, there is evidence to suggest that protein and/or amino acid ingestion prior to exercise can already stimulate MPS during exercise, thereby contributing to the muscle protein synthetic response to exercise [71, 72].

Ingestion of EAA in the period immediately after resistance exercise increases mTOR activation and MPS more than EAA or resistance exercise alone [1, 70, 73–75]. The result is that consuming protein within the first 2 h after resistance type exercise results in greater muscle hypertrophy and strength gains than consuming the same protein later [76, 77]. A similar increase in intracellular leucine content, mTOR signaling and MPS is seen when EAA are taken during endurance exercise [78]. However, as discussed above, the increase in protein synthesis after endurance exercise likely reflects myofibrillar and not mitochondrial protein synthesis [5]. Overall, these data suggest that athletes maintain bodyweight and muscle mass and promote protein turnover simply by consuming a calorie-neutral diet with supplemental protein timed for the first 30 min after a workout. This strategy can also be used to reduce lean body mass loss during periods of weight reduction [79].

Protein Quality and the Adaptation to Exercise

The data presented above suggest that consuming 20–25 g protein immediately following resistance exercise maximizes the mixed muscle protein synthetic response. However, the question remains which proteins are best for maximizing the response. Following ingestion, dietary protein is digested and absorbed [80]. Approximately 95% of amino acids are absorbed through the intestinal wall and released into the portal vein or used by the gut [81] with only ~50–60% of the ingested dietary protein being released into the systemic circulation [64, 82–84]. Depending on the protein quality, amount and the macronutrients ingested with the protein, the digestion and absorption kinetics can be modulated, resulting in more or less amino acids derived from that dietary protein being released in the circulation [85].

The most obvious example of how protein absorption can alter the MPS after exercise is seen between the two protein fractions, the so-called 'fast' and 'slow' proteins, found in milk [86]. The 'fast' protein is the acid soluble whey fraction that is rapidly absorbed and results in a dramatic rise in amino acid levels [74, 87–89]. The 'slow' protein is the acid-insoluble fraction consisting primarily of casein. When casein is ingested, the acidic environment of the stomach causes the protein to clump, slowing its passage from the stomach and absorption from the small intestine. The result is a modest, but prolonged increase in amino acids in the blood [74]. When consumed after a bout of resistance exercise, the rapidly absorbed whey stimulates protein synthesis to a greater degree than an isocaloric/isonitrogenous amount of the slower absorbed casein [74]. Hydrolyzing the casein to make it water soluble increases its absorption and the subsequent rate of MPS in response to an isonitrogenous amount of casein [90, 91], suggesting that the rate of absorption and uptake of amino acids results in different acute rates of protein synthesis [82]. However, the speed of absorption is not the only consideration. Soy protein, another acid-soluble 'fast' protein, does not stimulate MPS following resistance exercise to the same extent as whey [92], suggesting that the amount of leucine in the blood following ingestion may also play a role in stimulating MPS [93]. The latter is supported by the observation that even a more rapidly digested casein hydrolysate does not stimulate postprandial MPS to the extent as observed following the ingestion of whey protein [90]. The greater postprandial muscle protein synthetic response was significantly correlated with the postprandial rise in circulating plasma leucine concentrations. Therefore, the muscle protein synthetic response to dietary protein depends on the digestion and absorption kinetics as well as the amino acid composition of the protein.

Macronutrient Coingestion and Adaptation

Since the rate of amino acid appearance in the blood, with leucine in particular, is a key determinant of the MPS response, then a mixed meal of protein together with fat and carbohydrate may alter the postprandial muscle protein synthetic response. Consuming carbohydrates with protein slows amino acid uptake from the gut but also lowers liver amino acid uptake and gluconeogenesis [81, 94], suggesting a modest effect of carbohydrate on amino acid appearance in the blood. Even though fat consumption slows gastric emptying [95], coingestion of fat with protein does not seem to alter amino acid uptake kinetics [94]. In fact, when whole milk was directly compared with non-fat milk, the rate of amino acid uptake was found to be higher following resistance exercise in the presence of fat [96]. It remains to be determined how the postprandial muscle protein synthetic response can be modulated through the coingestion of other macronutrients. Besides the impact of fat and carbohydrate on protein digestion and absorption kinetics, the subsequent postprandial rise in circulating insulin may modulate muscle perfusion, thereby increasing amino acid delivery and/or amino acid uptake in skeletal muscle tissue. However, the effects of insulinogenic supplements (high in carbohydrate or arginine) have yet to be extensively tested.

Conclusion

Protein uptake, especially the amino acid leucine, into muscle results in the activation of mTOR and a subsequent increase in MPS. Following exercise, this results in an increase in the rate of myofibrillar protein synthesis and shifts muscle into a positive protein balance. However, it is important to note that protein consumption during acute post-exercise recovery does not seem to stimulate mitochondrial protein synthesis rates. Protein ingestion following exercise facilitates the increase in skeletal MPS rates following exercise, supporting muscle repair, growth and remodeling. For the strength athlete, exercise training increases the sensitivity to amino acids for at least 24 h after exercise, but immediate consumption of 20–25 g of rapidly absorbed protein will enhance MPS rates and drive the skeletal muscle hypertrophic response. At rest, 20–25 g of dietary protein should be consumed every 4–5 h and another 20–40 g prior to bedtime to facilitate the postprandial muscle protein synthetic response. In this way, consuming dietary protein can complement intense exercise training and facilitate the skeletal muscle adaptive response.

Disclosure Statement

N. Aguirre has no disclosures; L.J.C. van Loon has received research grants from Danone Research BV, DSM Food Specialties, Dutch Sugar Foundation and GlaxoSmithKline; K. Baar has received research grants from Astra Zenica and the E. Baar Research Trust.

References

1 Wilkinson SB, Phillips SM, Atherton PJ, et al: Differential effects of resistance and endurance exercise in the fed state on signalling molecule phosphorylation and protein synthesis in human muscle. J Physiol 2008;586: 3701–3717.

2 Phillips SM, Tipton KD, Aarsland A, et al: Mixed muscle protein synthesis and breakdown after resistance exercise in humans. Am J Physiol 1997;273:E99–E107.

3 Biolo G, Maggi SP, Williams BD, et al: Increased rates of muscle protein turnover and amino acid transport after resistance exercise in humans. Am J Physiol 1995;268:E514–E520.

4 Tipton KD, Ferrando AA, Phillips SM, et al: Postexercise net protein synthesis in human muscle from orally administered amino acids. Am J Physiol 1999;276:E628–E634.

5 Breen L, Philp A, Witard OC, et al: The influence of carbohydrate-protein co-ingestion following endurance exercise on myofibrillar and mitochondrial protein synthesis. J Physiol 2011;589:4011–4025.

6 Chesley A, MacDougall JD, Tarnopolsky MA, et al: Changes in human muscle protein synthesis after resistance exercise. J Appl Physiol 1992;73:1383–1388.

7 MacDougall JD, Gibala MJ, Tarnopolsky MA, et al: The time course for elevated muscle protein synthesis following heavy resistance exercise. Can J Appl Physiol 1995;20:480–486.

8 Baar K, Esser K: Phosphorylation of p70(S6k) correlates with increased skeletal muscle mass following resistance exercise. Am J Physiol 1999;276:C120–C127.

9 Terzis G, Georgiadis G, Stratakos G, et al: Resistance exercise-induced increase in muscle mass correlates with p70S6 kinase phosphorylation in human subjects. Eur J Appl Physiol 2008;102:145–152.

10 Drummond MJ, Fry CS, Glynn EL, et al: Rapamycin administration in humans blocks the contraction-induced increase in skeletal muscle protein synthesis. J Physiol 2009;587:1535–1546.

11 Bodine SC, Stitt TN, Gonzalez M, et al: Akt/mTOR pathway is a crucial regulator of skeletal muscle hypertrophy and can prevent muscle atrophy in vivo. Nat Cell Biol 2001;3:1014–1019.

12 Goodman CA, Frey JW, Mabrey DM, et al: The role of skeletal muscle mTOR in the regulation of mechanical load-induced growth. J Physiol 2011;589:5485–5501.

13 MacKenzie MG, Hamilton DL, Murray JT, et al: mVps34 is activated following high-resistance contractions. J Physiol 2009;587:253–260.

14 Sengupta S, Peterson TR, Sabatini DM: Regulation of the mTOR complex 1 pathway by nutrients, growth factors, and stress. Mol Cell 2010;40:310–322.

15 Peterson TR, Laplante M, Thoreen CC, et al: DEPTOR is an mTOR inhibitor frequently overexpressed in multiple myeloma cells and required for their survival. Cell 2009;137:873–886.

16 Frias MA, Thoreen CC, Jaffe JD, et al: mSin1 is necessary for Akt/PKB phosphorylation, and its isoforms define three distinct mTORC2s. Curr Biol 2006;16:1865–1870.

17 Pearce LR, Huang X, Boudeau J, et al: Identification of Protor as a novel Rictor-binding component of mTOR complex-2. Biochem J 2007;405:513–522.

18 Sarbassov DD, Ali SM, Kim DH, et al: Rictor, a novel binding partner of mTOR, defines a rapamycin-insensitive and raptor-independent pathway that regulates the cytoskeleton. Curr Biol 2004;14:1296–1302.

19 Schalm SS, Fingar DC, Sabatini DM, Blenis J: TOS motif-mediated raptor binding regulates 4E-BP1 multisite phosphorylation and function. Curr Biol 2003;13:797–806.

20 Schalm SS, Blenis J: Identification of a conserved motif required for mTOR signaling. Curr Biol 2002;12:632–639.

21 Land SC, Tee AR: Hypoxia-inducible factor 1alpha is regulated by the mammalian target of rapamycin (mTOR) via an mTOR signaling motif. J Biol Chem 2007;282:20534–20543.

22 Fonseca BD, Smith EM, Lee VH, et al: PRAS40 is a target for mammalian target of rapamycin complex 1 and is required for signaling downstream of this complex. J Biol Chem 2007;282:24514–24524.

23 Oshiro N, Takahashi R, Yoshino K, et al: The proline-rich Akt substrate of 40 kDa (PRAS40) is a physiological substrate of mammalian target of rapamycin complex 1. J Biol Chem 2007;282:20329–20339.

24 Garcia-Martinez JM, Alessi DR: mTOR complex 2 (mTORC2) controls hydrophobic motif phosphorylation and activation of serum- and glucocorticoid-induced protein kinase 1 (SGK1). Biochem J 2008;416:375–385.

25 Wang X, Proud CG: The mTOR pathway in the control of protein synthesis. Physiology (Bethesda) 2006;21:362–369.

26 Raught B, Peiretti F, Gingras AC, et al: Phosphorylation of eucaryotic translation initiation factor 4B Ser422 is modulated by S6 kinases. EMBO J 2004;23:1761–1769.

27 Wang X, Li W, Williams M, et al: Regulation of elongation factor 2 kinase by p90(RSK1) and p70 S6 kinase. EMBO J 2001;20:4370–4379.

28 Chen YW, Nader GA, Baar KR, et al: Response of rat muscle to acute resistance exercise defined by transcriptional and translational profiling. J Physiol 2002;545:27–41.

29 Lee J, Moir RD, McIntosh KB, Willis IM: TOR signaling regulates ribosome and tRNA synthesis via LAMMER/Clk and GSK-3 family kinases. Mol Cell 2012;45:836–843.

30 Philp A, Hamilton DL, Baar K: Signals mediating skeletal muscle remodeling by resistance exercise: PI3-kinase independent activation of mTORC1. J Appl Physiol 2011;110:561–568.

31 Byfield MP, Murray JT, Backer JM: hVps34 is a nutrient-regulated lipid kinase required for activation of p70 S6 kinase. J Biol Chem 2005;280:33076–33082.

32 Han JM, Jeong SJ, Park MC, Kim G, et al: Leucyl-tRNA synthetase is an intracellular leucine sensor for the mTORC1-signaling pathway. Cell 2012;149:410–424.

33 Sancak Y, Peterson TR, Shaul YD, Lindquist RA, et al: The Rag GTPases bind raptor and mediate amino acid signaling to mTORC1. Science 2008;320:1496–1501.

34 Sancak Y, Bar-Peled L, Zoncu R, et al: Regulator-Rag complex targets mTORC1 to the lysosomal surface and is necessary for its activation by amino acids. Cell 2010;141:290–303.

35 Baird FE, Bett KJ, MacLean C, et al: Tertiary active transport of amino acids reconstituted by coexpression of System A and L transporters in Xenopus oocytes. Am J Physiol Endocrinol Metab 2009;297:E822–E829.

36 Kanai Y, Hediger MA: The glutamate/neutral amino acid transporter family SLC1: molecular, physiological and pharmacological aspects. Pflugers Arch 2004;447:469–479.

37 Bevington A, Brown J, Butler H, et al: Impaired system A amino acid transport mimics the catabolic effects of acid in L6 cells. Eur J Clin Invest 2002;32:590–602.

38 Hyde R, Hajduch E, Powell DJ, et al: Ceramide down-regulates System A amino acid transport and protein synthesis in rat skeletal muscle cells. FASEB 2005;19:461–463.

39 Drummond MJ, Fry CS, Glynn EL, et al: Skeletal muscle amino acid transporter expression is increased in young and older adults following resistance exercise. J Appl Physiol 2011;111:135–142.

40 Drummond MJ, Glynn EL, Fry CS, et al: An increase in essential amino acid availability upregulates amino acid transporter expression in human skeletal muscle. Am J Physiol Endocrinol Metab 2010;298:E1011–E1018.

41 Carter HN, Hood DA: Contractile activity-induced mitochondrial biogenesis and mTORC1. Am J Physiol Cell Physiol 2012;303:C540–C547.

42 Neto JC, Lira FS, de Mello MT, Santos RV: Importance of exercise immunology in health promotion. Amino Acids 2011;41:1165–1172.

43 Castell LM, Newsholme EA: The effects of oral glutamine supplementation on athletes after prolonged, exhaustive exercise. Nutrition 1997;13:738–742.

44 Castell LM, Poortmans JR, Leclercq R, et al: Some aspects of the acute phase response after a marathon race, and the effects of glutamine supplementation. Eur J Appl Physiol Occup Physiol 1997;75:47–53.

45 Parry-Billings M, Budgett R, Koutedakis Y, et al: Plasma amino acid concentrations in the overtraining syndrome: possible effects on the immune system. Med Sci Sports Exerc 1992;24:1353–1358.

46 Bassit RA, Sawada LA, Bacurau RF, et al: The effect of BCAA supplementation upon the immune response of triathletes. Med Sci Sports Exerc 2000;32:1214–1219.

47 dos Santos RV, Caperuto EC, de Mello MT, et al: Effect of exercise on glutamine synthesis and transport in skeletal muscle from rats. Clin Exp Pharmacol Physiol 2009;36:770–775.

48 dos Santos RV, Caperuto EC, de Mello MT, Costa Rosa LF: Effect of exercise on glutamine metabolism in macrophages of trained rats. Eur J Appl Physiol 2009;107:309–315.

49 Santos RV, Caperuto EC, Costa Rosa LF: Effects of acute exhaustive physical exercise upon glutamine metabolism of lymphocytes from trained rats. Life Sci 2007;80:573–578.

50 MacLean DA, Graham TE, Saltin B: Stimulation of muscle ammonia production during exercise following branched-chain amino acid supplementation in humans. J Physiol 1996;493:909–922.

51 Cury-Boaventura MF, Levada-Pires AC, Folador A, et al: Effects of exercise on leukocyte death: prevention by hydrolyzed whey protein enriched with glutamine dipeptide. Eur J Appl Physiol 2008;103:289–294.

52 Sinclair LV, Finlay D, Feijoo C, et al: Phosphatidylinositol-3-OH kinase and nutrient-sensing mTOR pathways control T lymphocyte trafficking. Nat Immunol 2008;9:513–521.

53 Lagranha CJ, Hirabara SM, Curi R, Pithon-Curi TC: Glutamine supplementation prevents exercise-induced neutrophil apoptosis and reduces p38 MAPK and JNK phosphorylation and p53 and caspase 3 expression. Cell Biochem Funct 2007;25:563–569.

54 Lagranha CJ, Senna SM, de Lima TM, et al: Beneficial effect of glutamine on exercise-induced apoptosis of rat neutrophils. Med Sci Sports Exerc 2004;36:210–217.

55 Gleeson M: Dosing and efficacy of glutamine supplementation in human exercise and sport training. J Nutr 2008;138:2045S–2049S.

56 Trumbo P, Schlicker S, Yates AA, Poos M: Dietary reference intakes for energy, carbohydrate, fiber, fat, fatty acids, cholesterol, protein and amino acids. J Am Diet Assoc 2002;102:1621–1630.

57 Rodriguez NR, DiMarco NM, Langley S: Position of the American Dietetic Association, Dietitians of Canada, and the American College of Sports Medicine: nutrition and athletic performance. J Am Diet Assoc 2009;109: 509–527.

58 Tarnopolsky MA, Atkinson SA, MacDougall JD, et al: Evaluation of protein requirements for trained strength athletes. J Appl Physiol 1992;73:1986–1995.

59 Tarnopolsky MA, MacDougall JD, Atkinson SA: Influence of protein intake and training status on nitrogen balance and lean body mass. J Appl Physiol 1988;64:187–193.

60 Cuthbertson D, Smith K, Babraj J, et al: Anabolic signaling deficits underlie amino acid resistance of wasting, aging muscle. FASEB J 2005;19:422–424.

61 Moore DR, Robinson MJ, Fry JL, et al: Ingested protein dose response of muscle and albumin protein synthesis after resistance exercise in young men. Am J Clin Nutr 2009;89:161–168.

62 Burd NA, West DW, Moore DR, et al: Enhanced amino acid sensitivity of myofibrillar protein synthesis persists for up to 24 h after resistance exercise in young men. J Nutr 2011;141:568–573.

63 Yang Y, Churchward-Venne TA, Burd NA, et al: Myofibrillar protein synthesis following ingestion of soy protein isolate at rest and after resistance exercise in elderly men. Nutr Metab 2012;9:57.

64 Pennings B, Groen B, de Lange A, et al: Amino acid absorption and subsequent muscle protein accretion following graded intakes of whey protein in elderly men. Am J Physiol Endocrinol Metab 2012;302:E992–E999.

65 Tremblay F, Marette A: Amino acid and insulin signaling via the mTOR/p70 S6 kinase pathway. A negative feedback mechanism leading to insulin resistance in skeletal muscle cells. J Biol Chem 2001;276:38052–38060.

66 Bohe J, Low JF, Wolfe RR, Rennie MJ: Latency and duration of stimulation of human muscle protein synthesis during continuous infusion of amino acids. J Physiol 2001;532: 575–579.

67 Moore DR, Tang JE, Burd NA, et al: Differential stimulation of myofibrillar and sarcoplasmic protein synthesis with protein ingestion at rest and after resistance exercise. J Physiol 2009;587:897–904.

68 Groen BB, Res PT, Pennings B, et al: Intragastric protein administration stimulates overnight muscle protein synthesis in elderly men. Am J Physiol Endocrinol Metab 2012; 302:E52–E60.

69 Res PT, Groen B, Pennings B, et al: Protein ingestion prior to sleep improves post-exercise overnight recovery. Med Sci Sports Exerc 2012;44:1560–1569.

70 Tipton KD, Rasmussen BB, Miller SL, et al: Timing of amino acid-carbohydrate ingestion alters anabolic response of muscle to resistance exercise. Am J Physiol Endocrinol Metab 2001;281:E197–E206.

71 Koopman R, Pannemans DL, Jeukendrup AE, et al: Combined ingestion of protein and carbohydrate improves protein balance during ultra-endurance exercise. Am J Physiol Endocrinol Metab 2004;287:E712–E720.

72 Beelen M, Zorenc A, Pennings B, et al: Impact of protein coingestion on muscle protein synthesis during continuous endurance type exercise. Am J Physiol Endocrinol Metab 2011;300:E945–E954.

73 Coffey VG, Moore DR, Burd NA, et al: Nutrient provision increases signalling and protein synthesis in human skeletal muscle after repeated sprints. Eur J Appl Physiol 2011;111: 1473–1483.

74 West DW, Burd NA, Coffey VG, et al: Rapid aminoacidemia enhances myofibrillar protein synthesis and anabolic intramuscular signaling responses after resistance exercise. Am J Clin Nutr 2011;94:795–803.

75 Dreyer HC, Drummond MJ, Pennings B, et al: Leucine-enriched essential amino acid and carbohydrate ingestion following resistance exercise enhances mTOR signaling and protein synthesis in human muscle. Am J Physiol Endocrinol Metab 2008;294:E392–E400.

76 Andersen LL, Tufekovic G, Zebis MK, et al: The effect of resistance training combined with timed ingestion of protein on muscle fiber size and muscle strength. Metabolism 2005;54:151–156.

77 Esmarck B, Andersen JL, Olsen S, et al: Timing of postexercise protein intake is important for muscle hypertrophy with resistance training in elderly humans. J Physiol 2001; 535:301–311.

78 Pasiakos SM, McClung HL, McClung JP, et al: Leucine-enriched essential amino acid supplementation during moderate steady state exercise enhances postexercise muscle protein synthesis. Am J Clin Nutr 2011;94:809–818.

79 Mettler S, Mitchell N, Tipton KD: Increased protein intake reduces lean body mass loss during weight loss in athletes. Med Sci Sports Exerc 2010;42:326–337.

80 Jahan-Mihan A, Luhovyy BL, El Khoury D, Anderson GH: Dietary proteins as determinants of metabolic and physiologic functions of the gastrointestinal tract. Nutrients 2011;3: 574–603.

81 Deutz NE, Ten Have GA, Soeters PB, Moughan PJ: Increased intestinal amino-acid retention from the addition of carbohydrates to a meal. Clin Nutr 1995;14:354–364.

82 Koopman R, Crombach N, Gijsen AP, et al: Ingestion of a protein hydrolysate is accompanied by an accelerated in vivo digestion and absorption rate when compared with its intact protein. Am J Clin Nutr 2009;90:106–115.

83 Pennings B, Koopman R, Beelen M, et al: Exercising before protein intake allows for greater use of dietary protein-derived amino acids for de novo muscle protein synthesis in both young and elderly men. Am J Clin Nutr 2011;93:322–331.

84 Koopman R, Walrand S, Beelen M, et al: Dietary protein digestion and absorption rates and the subsequent postprandial muscle protein synthetic response do not differ between young and elderly men. J Nutr 2009;139: 1707–1713.

85 Boirie Y, Dangin M, Gachon P, et al: Slow and fast dietary proteins differently modulate postprandial protein accretion. Proc Natl Acad Sci USA 1997;94:14930–14935.

86 Beaufrere B, Dangin M, Boirie Y: The 'fast' and 'slow' protein concept; in Fürst P, Young V (eds): Proteins, Peptides and Amino Acids in Enteral Nutrition. Nestlé Nutr Workshop Ser Clin Perform Prog. Vevey, Nestec/Basel, Karger, 2000, vol 3, pp 121–131, discussion 131–133.

87 Dangin M, Boirie Y, Guillet C, Beaufrere B: Influence of the protein digestion rate on protein turnover in young and elderly subjects. J Nutr 2002;132:3228S–3233S.

88 Rieu I, Balage M, Sornet C, et al: Increased availability of leucine with leucine-rich whey proteins improves postprandial muscle protein synthesis in aging rats. Nutrition 2007; 23:323–331.

89 Tipton KD, Elliott TA, Cree MG, et al: Ingestion of casein and whey proteins result in muscle anabolism after resistance exercise. Med Sci Sports Exerc 2004;36:2073–2081.

90 Pennings B, Boirie Y, Senden JM, et al: Whey protein stimulates postprandial muscle protein accretion more effectively than do casein and casein hydrolysate in older men. Am J Clin Nutr 2011;93:997–1005.

91 Dideriksen KJ, Reitelseder S, Petersen SG, et al: Stimulation of muscle protein synthesis by whey and caseinate ingestion after resistance exercise in elderly individuals. Scand J Med Sci Sports 2011;21:e372–e383.

92 Tang JE, Moore DR, Kujbida GW, et al: Ingestion of whey hydrolysate, casein, or soy protein isolate: effects on mixed muscle protein synthesis at rest and following resistance exercise in young men. J Appl Physiol 2009; 107:987–992.

93 Norton LE, Wilson GJ, Layman DK, et al: Leucine content of dietary proteins is a determinant of postprandial skeletal muscle protein synthesis in adult rats. Nutr Metab 2012; 9:67.

94 Gaudichon C, Mahe S, Benamouzig R, et al: Net postprandial utilization of [15N]-labeled milk protein nitrogen is influenced by diet composition in humans. J Nutr 1999;129: 890–895.

95 Woodward ER: The mechanism by which ingested fat delays gastric emptying. Surgery 1957;41:1016–1018.

96 Elliot TA, Cree MG, Sanford AP, et al: Milk ingestion stimulates net muscle protein synthesis following resistance exercise. Med Sci Sports Exerc 2006;38:667–674.

van Loon LJC, Meeusen R (eds): Limits of Human Endurance.
Nestlé Nutr Inst Workshop Ser, vol 76, pp 103–120, (DOI: 10.1159/000350263)
Nestec Ltd., Vevey/S. Karger AG., Basel, © 2013

National Nutritional Programs for the 2012 London Olympic Games: A Systematic Approach by Three Different Countries

Louise M. Burke[a] · Nanna L. Meyer[b] · Jeni Pearce[c]

[a]Sports Nutrition, Australian Institute of Sport, Bruce, ACT, Australia; [b]University of Colorado and United States Olympic Committee, Colorado Springs, CO, USA; [c]Performance Nutrition, English Institute of Sport, Manchester, UK

Abstract

Preparing a national team for success at major sporting competitions such as the Olympic Games has become a systematic and multi-faceted activity. Sports nutrition contributes to this success via strategic nutritional interventions that optimize the outcomes from both the training process and the competitive event. This review summarizes the National Nutrition Programs involved with the 2012 London Olympic Games preparation of the Australian, British and American sports systems from the viewpoints of three key agencies: the Australian Institute of Sport, the English Institute of Sport and the United States Olympic Committee. Aspects include development of a nutrition network involving appropriately qualified sports dietitians/nutritionists within a multi-disciplinary team, recognition of continual updates in sports nutrition knowledge, and a systematic approach to service delivery, education and research within the athlete's daily training environment. Issues of clinical nutrition support must often be integrated into the performance nutrition matrix. Food service plays an important role in the achievement of nutrition goals during the Olympic Games, both through the efforts of the Athlete Dining Hall and catering activities of the host Olympic Games Organizing Committees as well as adjunct facilities often provided by National Olympic Committees for their own athletes.

Introduction

The achievement of success at the Olympic Games has become such a matter of national pride that many countries now undertake a systematic approach to the preparation of their teams through activities such as direct athlete support, establishment of sports institutes and specialized training centers, funding of sports science and sports medicine programs and assistance to National Sporting Organizations to achieve sound governance and performance plans. Sports nutrition is now recognized as an important branch of sports science/medicine that can promote sporting success via strategic nutritional interventions that optimize the outcomes from the training process and then reduce/delay the onset of various physiological factors that would otherwise limit competition performance.

The aim of this review is to showcase key areas in which nutrition programs can assist the preparation of Olympic athletes. It draws on the experiences of three separate countries with developed sports systems that incorporate an evidence-based approach to sports nutrition underpinned by the work of qualified sports dietitians and sports nutritionists. Experiences involved in the preparation for the 2012 London Olympic Games by the Australian, British and American sports systems will be provided by sports dietitians who were involved with Olympic programs from three key agencies: the Australian Institute of Sport (AIS), the English Institute of Sport and the United States Olympic Committee (USOC).

Implementation of Updated Knowledge in Sports Nutrition

The science and practice of sports nutrition is continually evolving, aided by an enthusiastic research base, the publication of peer-reviewed journals dedicated to sports nutrition and the development of consensus statements from expert groups such as the International Olympic Committee (IOC) and American College of Sports Medicine. A sports nutrition program should aim to both keep abreast of, and contribute to, such knowledge by taking the results of cutting edge research, undertaking further refinements to adapt it to specific events, conditions and individual athletes, and then developing systems that allow it to be practiced in the field. Table 1 summarizes some of the areas in which nutrition knowledge and practice has advanced over the last Olympiad; the examples include strategies which are new (e.g. nitrate supplementation), refinements of previously held ideas (e.g. guidelines for carbohydrate intake during competitive events) or simply a best response to an issue that has become more topical (e.g. treatment and prevention of illness and injury).

A systematic sports nutrition program should be underpinned by a strategic plan that clearly identifies core issues, and in particular targets those areas in which a worthwhile performance advantage may be gained. These areas may be determined by special challenges associated with the Olympic environment (e.g. heat, humidity, pollution), background expertise and resources, identification of existing nutrition problems or failure to engage in evidence-based practices, specific issues associated with events in which talented athletes are competing, and an assessment of the likely benefits afforded by new or improved dietary strategies. Programs developed by each country are likely to share some common elements but may also differ in other target areas.

Developing Systems to Provide a National Sports Nutrition Program

Various countries have developed a national approach to sports nutrition targeting the preparation and support of Olympic athletes. Different models include the development of nutrition programs within sports institutes (e.g. Australia, England, Wales, Scotland, Northern Ireland, New Zealand and Japan) or the support of programs by National Olympic Committees (e.g. America and Norway). The specific model will be developed to suit the unique characteristics, aims and funding avenues of the host country. Common threads to these programs include:

- engagement of appropriately qualified and experienced sports nutrition professionals (sports dietitians, sports nutritionists)
- development of specialized sports nutrition expertise that is sports specific and/or theme specific (e.g. weight-making, injury rehabilitation, altitude training)
- a mission or governing principles of performance enhancement and of being world class
- systematic programs for evidence-based best practice and quality control
- supportive links with a multi-disciplinary team
- strong career pathways including mentorship of junior staff and internships
- research and innovation programs
- strong ties with peak professional bodies for the training and promotion of sports dietitians/sports nutritionists
- collegiality with international counterparts and engagement with global networks

The three main outputs of these programs are education, research and athlete service delivery with services including dietary counseling on clinical and performance issues, hydration monitoring, nutrition support for team travel, facilitation of competition nutrition strategies, classes for cooking and nutrition life skills, and advice on supplement use. Some countries have developed specific activities to integrate education, research and service delivery around a single theme or framework. For example, the Sports Supplement Program of the AIS was established in 2000 as a holistic approach to supplement use by athletes within its own system. The Program provides state-of-the-art information on

Table 1. Key areas of new sports nutrition knowledge and practice since 2008 for implementation at London Olympic Games 2012

Issue	Overview
Areas of updated knowledge with good evidence base leading to new practice guidelines	
Optimal protein synthesis in acute recovery after exercise for muscle hypertrophy, adaptation and repair	Intake of 20–25 g of high-quality protein close to exercise, particularly from rapidly digesting protein-rich foods, optimizes muscle protein synthesis after exercise [12, 13]
Carbohydrate intake during brief high-intensity exercise lasting ~1 h	Regular intake of small amounts of carbohydrate, including mouth rinsing, enhances pacing and performance probably through direct stimulation of central nervous system by carbohydrate-sensing receptors in oral cavity [14]
Carbohydrate intake during prolonged exercise lasting >2 h	During prolonged events (>2.5–3 h), there is evidence of a dose response to performance effects of carbohydrate intake with optimal outcomes being achieved by intakes of up to 80–90 g/h [15] Maximal rates of oxidation of carbohydrates ingested during exercise are achieved by using mixtures of sugars that are absorbed from the intestines using different transport mechanisms (e.g. glucose + fructose) [16] Capacity for oxidation of exogenous carbohydrate during exercise is increased by chronic practice with consuming carbohydrate during exercise [17]
New areas with fast-tracked interest	
Acute supplementation with nitrate/ beetroot juice	Intake of a source of nitrate (found in beetroot juice among another sources) in the 2 h (and perhaps days) prior to an exercise test may enhance exercise economy and performance [18, 19], although results are less apparent in higher caliber athletes [19]
Monitoring and maintaining optimal vitamin D status	Athletes represent a subgroup at risk of suboptimal vitamin D status; vitamin D is important for optimal function of many body systems including bone health, muscle function and immune system [20]
Areas of continued gathering of evidence base but requiring further work	
'Training low' with carbohydrates to enhance adaptive response to exercise stimulus	Training with low glycogen content (by doing a second workout soon after a glycogen depleting session) or training in a fasted state amplifies many signaling pathways responsible for training adaptations, especially those involved in fat oxidation [21, 22]; since the potential downside of such training is a reduction in exercise intensity, it needs to be considered as a periodized rather than universal training model [22]
Chronic supplementation with β-alanine	Supplementation with 200–400 g β-alanine, spread as 3–6 g/day over 4–10 weeks will increase muscle carnosine content [23] Increased carnosine content increases muscle buffering capacity and perhaps other muscle functions which may lead to enhanced performance [24]
Low-dose caffeine supplementation including intake during events	Supplementation with 3 mg/kg caffeine before or during exercise, including just before the onset of fatigue enhances performance of many types of sports via effects on central nervous system [25]
Combining the use of supplements which may individually enhance performance	Supplements such as caffeine, bicarbonate, nitrate, β-alanine and creatine which may individually enhance the performance of an event may have additive or interactive effects when used together [2]

Examples of targeted events on Olympic Program	Practical implementation for specific athletes or situations
Resistance exercise and key/quality training sessions Events which require repeated races/matches	Athletes should plan their meals and snacks to allow an even spread of moderate amounts of high-quality protein over the day, including after key workouts/events
Sustained events of ~1 h – Cycling time trial – 20 km race walk (Possibly) triathlon (Possibly) team sports – football, handball, basketball, hockey, volleyball and water polo (Possibly) to rescue reduced training capacity during 'train low' strategies (see below)	According to the logistics of their event, the athlete should experiment with regularly swilling, sucking or consuming carbohydrate sources such as sports drinks, gels or confectionery with a focus on promoting mouth contact with the carbohydrate
Longer distance events – Cycling road race – Marathon – 50 km race walking	During prolonged races, a well-practiced race plan should attempt to deliver carbohydrate at rates of up to 80–90 g/h from a range of sources of 'multiple transportable carbohydrates' including specialized sports products Practice in training should help to fine tune the race plan as well as achieve adaptations (probably in the gut) to increase capacity for muscle oxidation of carbohydrates consumed during exercise
Sustained high-intensity events lasting 1–8 min (e.g. swimming, rowing, middle distance athletics, track cycling, canoe/kayak) (Possibly) team sports (see above) (Possibly) sustained events of ~1 h (see above), triathlon and longer distance events (see above)	The athlete might benefit from experimenting with supplementation of beetroot juice or other sources providing ~300 mg nitrate in the hours prior to an event, perhaps supported by intake in days beforehand. Future research is warranted to determine the range of events in which this might be useful, and optimal protocols of use
Athletes at risk of low exposure to UVB in sunlight (e.g. athletes who train indoors or have minimal exposure to sunshine within middle of day, live in latitudes >35°, have dark skin, remain covered or with sunscreen when outdoors)	Athletes at risk of low UVB exposure should be regularly screened and receive appropriate vitamin D supplementation if status is found to be suboptimal
(Possibly) training for – Sustained high-intensity events (see above) – Team sports (see above) – Sustained events of ~1 h (see above) – Triathlon and prolonged distance events	Training sessions undertaken with low carbohydrate availability (low glycogen, or overnight fasted) might be deliberately scheduled into the periodized training calendar to take advantage of the enhanced stimulus of some training adaptations; the value of such training will vary according to the sport and the individual athlete's response
Sustained high-intensity events lasting 1–8 min (see above) (Possibly) team sports (see above) (Possibly) interval training	The athlete might benefit from experimenting with 4–10 weeks' supplementation providing a total intake of 200–400 g β-alanine; future research is warranted to determine the range of events in which this might be useful, and optimal protocols of use
Triathlon and prolonged-distance events (see above) Sustained events of ~1 h (see above) Sustained high-intensity events lasting 1–8 min (see above) Team sports (see above) Sports involving repeated bouts/races (e.g. multisport track and field; martial arts)	The athlete might benefit from experimenting with low doses of caffeine (3 mg/kg total) including intake during and late in the event Future research is warranted to determine the range of events in which this might be useful; individual experimentation is warranted to find optimal protocols of use
Sustained high-intensity events (e.g. swimming, rowing, middle distance athletics, track cycling, canoe/kayak) Team sports (see above) Triathlon and sustained events of ~1 h (see above) Longer distance events (see above)	The athlete might benefit from experimenting with the combined use of supplements that are known, individually, to enhance the performance of their event; careful experimentation is required to account for interactive effects; future research is warranted to determine the range of events in which this might be useful, and optimal protocols of use

Table 1. Continued

Issue	Overview
Areas of high priority requiring a response despite small evidence base	
Reducing illness risk with general dietary support and use of immune-enhancing dietary factors	Inadequate energy and carbohydrate availability reduces immune system function [26] There is some evidence that some immune-enhancing nutrients can reduce the risk of contracting illness (e.g. probiotics, polyphenols) or reduce the impact of an illness once it is contracted (e.g. zinc) [26]
Enhancing rehabilitation with proactive nutrition support	Adequate energy availability and a good spread of high-quality protein are required to support injury repair and minimize the atrophy associated with disuse [3] Other nutrients may be useful for promoting injury rehabilitation or reducing disuse atrophy (e.g. fish oils, creatine) [3]
Areas of dispute or controversy	
Importance of hydration during events	There has been recent publicity of the view that hydration/dehydration is not important in performance outcomes and that athletes need only drink during sporting events if they are thirsty [27]; this is at odds with information that few events in elite sport offer athletes the opportunity for ad libitum fluid intake to address thirst

the use of supplements and sports foods, targets sport-specific research in this area and manages the provision of products that are at low risk of causing an inadvertent doping outcome due to contamination with substances that are prohibited by the World Anti-Doping Agency [1]. Sports foods and supplements are classified into 4 different categories based on the currently available evidence of their efficacy in performance enhancement and risk of doping outcomes [2].

A feature of the Program is a website (www.ausport.gov.au/ais/nutrition/supplements) providing continually updated resources on the classification system, as well as fact sheets and summaries of available research on products within group A (sound evidence for specific uses in sport and considered for provision for use by AIS athletes) and group B (prioritized for research and provided to AIS athletes under a research protocol). The strategic decision to make these resources freely available was taken to promote the expertise of the AIS on this topic and thus build credibility with its own athletes. Other benefits include maintaining transparency requirements of a taxpayer-funded organization and being accessible to AIS athletes in a variety of locations. However, the recent development of a separate and enhanced version, on a secure website available only to sports scientists within the Australian system, has allowed discussion forums and the dissemination of unpublished research and specific protocols for obtaining and using supplements and sports foods within the AIS and wider Australian sports systems. In this way, a competitive edge can be achieved while maintaining the original objectives of the program.

Examples of targeted events on Olympic Program	Practical implementation for specific athletes or situations
Athletes or situations at high risk of illness	The athlete should be proactive with strategies that provide adequate energy and carbohydrate availability During periods of high volume/intensity training or in high-risk environments, the athlete might benefit from experimenting with immune-enhancing nutrients; future research is warranted to determine the range of substances which might be useful, and optimal protocols of use
Athletes incurring significant injuries, especially those undergoing surgery or major alteration of training	The athlete should work with his/her sports nutritionist to implement an energy- and protein-adequate diet to support injury repair during acute and longer term rehabilitation Further research is warranted to determine other nutrients and substances that can reduce the atrophy associated with disuse and enhance injury repair
Team sports (see above) Triathlon Sustained events of ~1 h (see above) Longer distance events (see above) 20 and 50 km race walks Cycling time trial and road race	Each athlete should develop an individualized event nutrition plan which balances the specific opportunities provided by the event to consume foods or drinks, the potential benefits of intake of fluid, carbohydrate and other ingredients, and individual tolerance and experiences

The establishment of a strong, sustainable National Nutrition Program is a long-term goal which can be challenged by fluctuations in funding resources, changes in models of sports administration and the ability to obtain qualified and skilled staff. Both a function of, and an aid to, the maintenance of such a program is formal and informal collaboration with other organizations and global networks (e.g. Professionals in Nutrition for Exercise and Sport: PINES) with similar goals for developing and enhancing the discipline on an international level. The sharing of expertise and experiences within these networks allows the development of international projects (e.g. development of catering guidelines for major sporting events, production of global education resources) and the rapid deployment of information (e.g. the identification of contaminated supplements and foods).

Dealing with Clinical Nutrition Needs of Athletes

Although sports nutrition programs are primarily focused on dietary strategies to optimize performance, in many cases athletes must also deal with nutrition issues related to health and well-being, including the risk of illness and injury arising from their sports pursuits. Athletes at all levels become injured due to heavy training load, overuse, contact/impact, illness and physical/biomechanical challenges or irregularities. Several programs have targeted specific resources to reduce the development of injuries and/or promote rehabilitation of existing problems underpinned by evidence-based nutrition strategies [3]. One example of this is the Intensive Rehabilitation Unit established as a collaboration of the English Institute of Sport and the British Olympic Association. This unit was designed to provide consistent, integrated and intensive rehabilitation in an environment that optimizes recovery and promotes the return to training and performance. The focus of the Intensive Rehabilitation Unit is to reduce the number of lost training days and to assist athletes to return to full training in a realistic and responsible time frame. Nutrition services are a key component of the multidisciplinary team outputs, with the sports nutritionist attending case reviews and contributing to integrated intervention and management plans. Highly individualized rehabilitation nutrition advice is provided in consultation with the multi-disciplinary team members, with information being delivered back to the sport-specific sports dietitians and performance nutritionists on discharge. An additional benefit of the unit is to provide an opportunity to work with athletes from sports which lack the services of sports dietitians/performance nutritionist and thus promote the discipline to highly receptive athletes, coaches and sports science/medicine staff.

Over the years, an increasingly large number of athletes with clinical nutrition issues have reached the elite levels in sport (and won gold medals). These conditions which require a delicate balance of integration of management within a performance nutrition matrix include insulin-dependent diabetes [4] and, more recently, a wider range of food allergies and intolerance which range in severity from mild discomfort to anaphylactic shock. Special food needs must be included in the catering arrangements for training camps and international sporting events. While a single sport training camp provides an environment in which these measures can be tightly controlled and easily monitored, this becomes more difficult as the number of athletes and special needs increase. For example, at the multisport 'holding camp' undertaken immediately prior to the 2012 Games by the British Olympic Association, 13 different food allergens were identified as requiring strict labeling and menu scheduling. The components which were monitored ranged from the more common (e.g. gluten, lactose, dairy, soy, wheat, general nut and shellfish) allergens to the lesser known (e.g. nut-specific allergens in walnut, hazelnut, brazil nut and sesame seeds, spices including cinnamon, and individual fruit and vegetables). The clinical skills of a sports dietitian were required to work with the catering team to identify the presence or contamination of an allergen in various foods, and to establish a uniform labeling system for menu choices. Menus must also incorporate a range of options for strict vegans, a range of vegetarian styles, and religious requests from halal to kosher.

Ramadan – A Special Challenge of the London Olympics

A unique feature of the London Olympics was the coincidence of the competition calendar (July 27 to August 12, 2012) with the Islamic holy month of Ramadan (July 20 to August 18, 2012). Fasting during Ramadan, one of the five pillars of the Muslim faith, involves abstinence from all fluid and food intake during the period from first light to sunset, as well as rituals involved with breaking of the fast and various prayer and feasts throughout the night [5]. Actual fasting practices vary according to the individual, their cultural and religious environment, their geographical location, the changing dates of Ramadan and other factors such as work and family commitments. However, for Muslim athletes who chose to fast during the London Olympic period, the nutritional implications were likely to involve lengthy periods without nutrient intake and inflexibility with the timing of eating and drinking around a 24-hour period. Changes to usual dietary choices or performance nutrition goals may have also occurred due to the special foods involved with various cultural rituals. Each factor alters an athlete's ability to achieve their nutrition goals in different ways [6]. An immediate issue is the inability to consume important nutrients before, during or after a specific exercise session to support immediate needs of performance or recovery. Furthermore, athletes may be unable to consume the recommended pattern of nutrient intake over a day for optimal nutrient availability or, in the case where nutrient needs are substantially elevated, meet total daily needs from the restricted period available for eating.

The implications of the overlap between the London Olympics and Ramadan required several activities. First, catering for athletes, officials and the public at the Games was organized to ensure that appropriate foods were suitable for key meals such as *Iftar* (breaking of the fast in the evening) and *sohoor* (the last meal before dawn). Second, various agencies including the IOC and Federation Internationale de Football Association hosted activities to produce position statements [7] and education resources [7, 8] to guide Muslim athletes in making well-informed decisions about undertaking high-intensity sport in stressful conditions while fasting, and, if fasting, to develop a personalized plan underpinned by professional guidance. At the time of writing this paper, there were no data on the number of Muslim athletes who fasted while competing in the London Olympics.

Food Service at Olympic Summer Games

The history of food provision at the summer Olympic Games over the past century (1896–2012), as reviewed by Pelly et al. [9], provides an interesting perspective on the evolution of sport nutrition research and practice. The common belief in the early 1900s was that protein intake was linked to athleticism. This was reflected at the Paris 1924 Olympics, where a dining hall was included in the first communal accommodations; this served a variety of foods with the emphasis on meats, eggs, and cheeses. Even though studies demonstrating the role of dietary carbohydrates in increasing muscle glycogen and exercise endurance had been published by the late 1960s, it was not until the 1984 Olympic Games in Los Angeles that expert nutrition advice allowed these considerations to be reflected in the dining hall menu choices [9]. Product sponsorship, including partnerships with the food/beverage/sports food manufacturers and restaurant chains also became more evident at these Games. More recent developments in food provision at Olympic Games include the availability of low-fat, high-carbohydrate menu options (Atlanta, 1996), menu and food composition labeling using nutrition cards (Barcelona, 1992) and a nutrition kiosk and interactive website for athletes' questions, concerns, and guidance (Sydney, 2000) [9].

The outstanding challenge for the food service company which wins the catering bid for the Summer Olympic Games is to feed over 10,000 athletes from more than 200 countries over a continuous 24-hour cycle for a 20- to 25-day period. Meal provision must meet a variety of food preferences, including cultural and religious diversity, dietary restrictions, event-specific sports nutrition needs, and changes in nutrition needs between periods of final training, taper, competition and celebration. Food safety issues are of high priority, and healthy nutrition guidelines should also be taken into account. Information about the menu and individual food items should be provided to the end users via nutrition cards, websites and a nutrition kiosk. The integration of the expertise of sports nutritionists/dietitians in the development and implementation of the food service at the Summer Olympic Games is a relatively recent development. In fact, it was only after the Sydney Games in 2000, that the IOC mandated the requirement for a dietitian to collaborate with the successful catering company to ensure that nutritional, cultural, and religious dietary needs are accommodated [9].

At the London 2012 Olympic Games, the US-based catering company Aramark hired several dietitians to undertake this task, some of whom were specialized in sport nutrition. These sports dietitians established criteria for energy, macro- and micronutrient targets for menu items, based on the predicted physiological demands of various sports grouped into categories of endurance, strength and power, and precision (technical, aesthetic). A novel activity was the development of a web-based education tool to provide information on the menu structure and composition of individual food items [10]. An additional focus of the catering operation was to provide sustainable food of highest quality, with a code [11] to challenge food service providers and caterers to adopt, or further develop, practices that are environmentally sound, socially just and ethical. Personal communication with Aramark elicited that there was an additional time commitment required to assure that products met the code (e.g. Red Tractor certified, Free Range, Marine Conservation Society). There were also problems associated with the sourcing of sufficient locally available food supplies to provide 40,000 meals per day and over 1 million meals throughout the games.

The achievement of culturally appropriate meals within a performance-based menu for athletes from more than 200 countries is a major challenge for the food service provider for a global event like the Olympic Games. Here, the input of members of PINES has been well placed to provide assistance. In preparation for the Beijing Olympics in 2008, a working group of PINES circulated a survey that aimed to capture international food preferences at Olympic Games. The results of this survey initiated a systematic review process of the menus developed by the successful catering company, with the assistance of PINES being sought by the IOC. This process begins once the menu and concepts are written by the catering company and are passed on to the IOC by the local organizing committee to be reviewed by PINES. For the London 2012 Games, the PINES International Sports Nutrition and Catering Working Group received the menus in October 2011. The completion of the review occurred within a month, at which time point the London Organizing Committee for the Olympic Games, in conjunction with the catering company, addressed several of the raised concerns and questions which were subsequently communicated to PINES. The experience in London, however, as well as other past experiences suggest that not all concerns are addressed via this model; a commitment to review at the time of tender applications and again at the implementation from soft to hard Olympic Village opening should be sought in the future.

Alternative Food Service Facilities

Food service provision at the Olympic Games is typically focused on what is served in the Olympic Village and at the sporting venues. Although the majority of athletes reside in the Olympic Village, some athletes choose not to do so in the period prior to competition. Reasons include the management of distractions and communal living, the avoidance of attention (high-profile athletes) or large travel commitments between the Village and sporting venues, and the wish to provide a familiar surrounding within an environment that is otherwise unusual to the athlete. Some countries organize alternative accommodation and catering for various proportions of their team. For example, since the Atlanta

Games (1996), the USOC has committed to the creation of a High Performance Training Center (HPTC) within the Olympic host city, with this facility typically being integrated into the setting of a university. The aim of the HPTC is to establish a mini-training center and a familiar meal service that caters to 150–200 American athletes, coaches, and staff before and during the Games. The USOC food service team develops most of the performance-based menus but contracts a catering company to produce the food. Activities include reviewing bids from a variety of catering companies, interviewing executive and sous chefs, identifying the food chain, traceability, and delivery patterns, securing quantity, quality, and safety of food within a pre-set budget, and working with sponsors and leveraging on value-in-kind products for economical reasons. Depending on the country, other critical steps for on-site success include converting recipe units and testing the recipes with foreign products. Establishing HPTC dining services requires at least 12–18 months of preparation, and the on-site setup requires at least a 2- to 4-week period before the 'hard opening'. In the past, the HPTCs served around 17,000 meals through the Olympic Games.

Special Nutrition Services during the Olympic Games

Although the majority of activities in the nutritional preparation of elite athletes are undertaken during the training phase, assistance in team travel is now a recognized activity undertaken by sports dietitians and nutritionists. Indeed, many countries now include sports nutritional professionals within their Olympic Team, both in accredited and additional staff, to continue usual services to their specific sports or athletes and/or undertake a global role of nutrition services within the medical headquarters team. The numbers and roles of sports dietitians/nutritionists involved in the US, UK and Australian Olympic teams are summarized in figures 1–3. Activities undertaken by these professionals during the Games period include:

- assisting athletes with orientation and management of nutrition needs within the Olympic Dining Hall and catering facilities; liaising with nutrition services provided by Host City Organizing Committees
- facilitating food requirements for athletes with special nutrition needs
- organization and management of additional sports foods and products; oversight of nutritional supplementation protocols
- oversight and assistance with special nutrition strategies (e.g. pre-cooling strategies, recovery nutrition)
- assistance at feed zones in ultra-endurance events (road cycling, marathon, 50-km walk)

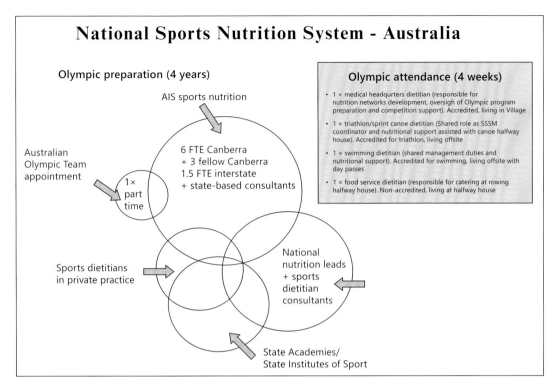

National Sports Nutrition System - Australia

Olympic preparation (4 years)

AIS sports nutrition

Australian
Olympic Team
appointment

1×
part
time

6 FTE Canberra
+ 3 fellow Canberra
1.5 FTE interstate
+ state-based consultants

Sports dietitians
in private practice

National
nutrition leads
+ sports
dietitian
consultants

State Academies/
State Institutes of Sport

Olympic attendance (4 weeks)

- 1 × medical headqurters dietitian (responsible for nutrition networks development, oversigh of Olympic program preparation and competition support). Accredited, living in Village

- 1 × triathlon/sprint canoe dietitian (Shared role as SSSM coordinator and nutritional support assisted with canoe halfway house). Accredited for triathlon, living offsite

- 1 × swimming dietitian (shared management duties and nutritional support). Accredited for swimming, living offsite with day passes

- 1 × food service dietitian (responsible for catering at rowing halfway house). Non-accredited, living at halfway house

Fig. 1. National nutrition system model in Australia.

- oversight of strategies of weight-making athletes
- individual education and counseling of athletes for acute and chronic issues
- oversight of nutrition monitoring activities (e.g. hydration monitoring)

Final Outcomes

The period after each Olympic Games is spent undertaking a review of the programs and services provided during the 4-year Olympiad and at the Games and the successes and failures of these activities. The highly publicized medal tallies are scrutinized on an absolute basis, and relative to factors such as the population base and the funding committed to Olympic or elite sports programs within each country. Some of the results of these reviews will become public access documents, while many countries maintain such records as internal communications. Each National Nutrition Program will undertake its own audit of achievements, success and failures, challenges and aids. Some of the immediate reflections from Nutrition Service Providers involved in the London Olympics

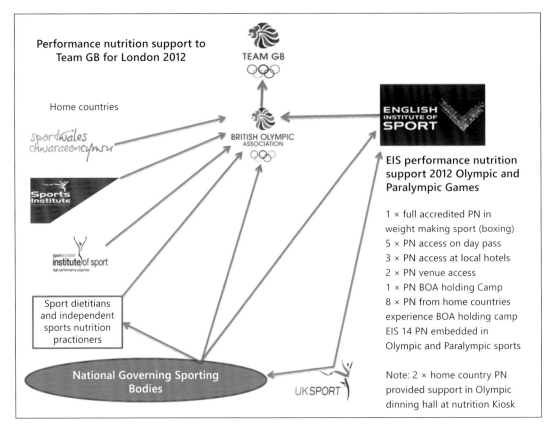

Fig. 2. National nutrition system model in Great Britain.

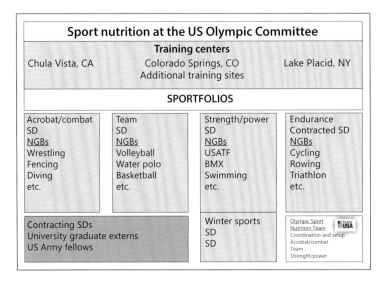

Fig. 3. National nutrition system model in United States of America. NGB = National Governing Body (sport); SD = sports dietitian.

Burke · Meyer · Pearce

Table 2. Reflections on experiences at the 2012 London Olympic Games

Country	Actual achievements		Reflections on most successful nutrition activities and positive experiences/characteristics	Reflections on challenges/difficulties
Australia	Gold	7	'Easy' Olympic schedule due to lack of environmental challenges, 'friendly' sports timetable: able to operate more effectively and cover more issues	Distraction due to publicity of specifically timed release of *British Medical Journal* articles criticizing sports food/supplement industry and sports nutrition research
	Silver	16		
	Bronze	12		
	Total	35	Excellent Olympic Games organization and facilities	
	Place	10th	Few episodes of illness	Difficulty in accessing special food needs in dining hall (gluten-free staples, combined allergen dairy/egg/gluten free)
	Comments	Below expectations and goals	Minimal impact of Ramadan: no fasting athletes in team	Lack of some everyday staples in dining hall (low fat dairy, bread)
			Nearby access to shopping center facilitated ability to obtain missing food supplies	Morale maintenance in light of below par performances and results (negative press from home and locally)
			Enhanced level of expertise of National Nutrition Network with organized mentoring AIS Sports Supplement Program: enhanced program due to targeted event-specific research program and secure Clearinghouse dissemination of information	Weight-making athletes: last minute requirements to lose large amounts of body mass (e.g. 4.8 kg in 1 day, 5 kg in 1 week) Indiscriminate supplement use by small handful of athletes 'outside' system
			Enhanced engagement in National Network (Nutrition Leads, Clearinghouse communication)	Poor engagement of some sports on research projects with high level athletes: research protocols diluted
			Successful implementation of halfway house at Eton-Dorney for rowing, sprint canoe/kayak Recovery center: conveniently located offsite to offer specialized recovery modalities Individual successes with new or improved nutrition strategies with some athletes	
Great Britain	Gold	29	'Business as usual' approach due to familiar venues, environmental conditions and Olympic menus	Distractions and pressures to perform from media, friends and family
	Silver	17		Implementing research project with time constraints and diluting the time availability of practitioners and athletes prior to Olympic Games
	Bronze	19	Performance nutritionist involved in local venue menu planning, on site in local hotel and on day passes to provide support, Sport-specific practitioners imbedded in sports and familiar sports science personnel around athletes and coaches at all times	
	Total	65		
	Place	3rd		Frustrations in finding daily menu items in Olympic village dining hall
	Comments	Outperformed targets	First full-time performance nutritionist accredited into the Olympic village in a weight-making sport	Lack of easily identifiable allergen-free foods (gluten-free breads) and confusion over label advice interpretation (free from or contains allergen)
			Front load professional performance nutritionist development in first 2 years after Beijing High focus on team and personal hygiene, familiar microbial environment	Sports performance food items (flavored milk) not available in Olympic dining hall Requests to start a supplement or to change a supplement dose in days leading into competition
			No impact of Ramadan due to early discussions and individual responses planned ahead Active supplement contamination free program with preferred supplement providers and bespoke product development and research support	Provision of high nutrient value liquid meals for facial injuries
			Support of dedicated specialist injury rehab center for elite athletes and philosophies in promoting return to training and active competition	
			Performance nutritionist from the four home countries and external nutritionist working collectively as one team at pre-Olympic camps and providing support during the Olympic Games High morale and positive focus on the organization and performance nutrition roles	

Table 2. Continued

Country	Actual achievements		Reflections on most successful nutrition activities and positive experiences/ characteristics	Reflections on challenges/difficulties
United States	Gold	46	Preparation and planning within USOC time consuming but effective (4 sports dietitians as part of Olympic team)	Logistics, transportation, traffic created difficulties for delivering boxed meals, packed recovery foods and fluids
	Silver	29	Sports dietitians worked effectively with sports	Difficulty keeping up with restocking recovery foods/fluids
	Bronze	29	HPTC met expected needs of athletes training/competing at nearby venues	Main village dining hall appeared overwhelming to athletes; difficulty navigating
	Total	104	Team USA Recovery Stations successfully implemented	Unresolved issues in village dining hall regarding nutrition cards, consistent labeling of allergens, procedures to avoid cross-contamination of allergens, exposure of foods without appropriate serving utensils or sneeze guards
	Place	1st	Contingency plans available and utilized	
	Comments	Met targets	Food provision in main village optimized; however, issues remained despite PINES and feedback to catering company by multiple NOC sports dietitians	Lack of food at venues within Olympic Park; LOCOG considered proximity of village main dining hall sufficient
			Food service company's website and kiosk effective for identification of foods for athletes with dietary restrictions	Field-based trials with performance-enhancing supplements always problematic with elite athletes

LOCOG = London Organising Committee of the Olympic and Paralympic Games.

Table 3. Summary of challenges and benefits of researching and implementing new nutrition strategies

Phase	Positives	Challenges
Research	Collecting information on elite, or at least highly trained, athletes adds crucial information on the general and event-specific evidence base underpinning use of a nutrition strategy in sport Athletes and coaches who participate in research studies gain direct evidence of their event-specific and individual response to a nutrition strategy Other benefits to athletes and coaches arise from involvement in research: enhanced relationship with sports scientist, appreciation of the research process and the development of an evidence base, enhanced training, identification of other suboptimal practices or issues that can be enhanced	Research is resource and time intensive and may not be included in standard sports budgets and timetables It is difficult to gain adequate access to the highest caliber athletes to undertake optimally designed research projects There are limited opportunities to alter existing training/nutrition programs or collect invasively derived data By definition, elite athletes are few in number; studies may be underpowered Many athletes and coaches do not appreciate the research process; even when they are engaged in a project, they may insist on changes that dilute the research design (e.g. poor standardization of diet or background training, allocation of treatment to the best athletes rather than random allocation; preference for observational research without placebo group or treatment) Athletes may develop career ending injuries and drop out of research or protocols
Implementation of new knowledge	Athletes benefit from an evidence-based nutrition strategy which directly enhances performance or allows them to achieve better training outcomes Addresses different athlete learning styles which dictate willingness to engage in new knowledge Athletes can receive a placebo effect, which also enhances performance, due to the extra confidence associated with having new or special strategies to implement	It is unlikely that research will be able to definitively identify ergogenic strategies for every specific event or individual athlete; some practices will need to be determined by intuition rather than direct evidence base It can be difficult to arrange supplies of new supplements or food products in the Olympic environment due to issues with international delivery (customs requirements), Village delivery (security requirements) issues or clashes with official sponsors

are summarized in table 2, with a final summary of the successes and failures specifically involved in gaining and interpreting the data from nutrition research activities being provided in table 3. It is anticipated that the next Olympiad through to the 2016 Rio de Janeiro will provide some clarification of current issues as well as introduce some totally novel ideas and practices.

Disclosure Statement

None of these authors has anything to declare.

References

1 Geyer H, Parr MK, Reinhart U, Schrader Y, Mareck U, Schanzer W: Analysis of non-hormonal nutritional supplements for anabolic-androgenic steroids – results of an international study. Int J Sports Med 2004;25: 124–129.

2 Burke LM, Broad L, Cox G, Desbrow B, Dziedzik C, Gurr S, Lalor B, Shaw G, Shaw N, Slater G: Dietary Supplements and Nutritional Ergogenic Aids; in Burke LM, Deakin V (eds): Clinical Sports Nutrition, ed 4. Sydney, McGraw-Hill, 2010, pp 419–500.

3 Burke LM, Maughan RJ: Nutrition and therapy; in Zachazewski J, Magee D (eds): IOC Handbook: Sports Therapy, in press.

4 Deakin V, Wilson D, Cooper G: Special Needs: Athletes with Diabetes; in Burke LM, Deakin V (eds): Clinical Sports Nutrition, ed 4. Sydney, McGraw-Hill, pp 578–601.

5 Zerguini Y, Ahmed QA, Dvorak J: The Muslim football player and Ramadan: current challenges. J Sports Sci 2012;30(suppl 1):S3–S7.

6 Burke LM, King C: Ramadan fasting and the goals of sports nutrition around exercise. J Sports Sci 2012;30(suppl 1):S21–S31.

7 Maughan RJ, Al-Kharusi W, Binnett MS, Budgett R, Burke LM, Coyle EF, Elwani R, Guezennec CY, Limna J, Mujika I, Ramadan J, Schamasch P, Shirreffs SM, Vennard P: Fasting and sports: a summary statement of the IOC workshop. Br J Sports Med 2012;46: 457.

8 Maughan RJ, Zerguini Y, Chalabi H, Dvorak J (eds): Ramadan and football. J Sports Sci 2012;(suppl 1):S1–S117.

9 Pelly FE, O'Connor HT, Denyer GS, Caterson ID: Evolution of food provision to athletes at the summer Olympic Games. Nutr Rev 2011;69:321–332.

10 http://www.london2012.com/documents/ locog-publications/food-vision.pdf; retrieved on March 13, 2012.

11 http://www.london2012.com/about-us/ publications/publication=locog-sustainable-sourcing-code/; retrieved June 5, 2012.

12 Churchward-Venne TA, Burd NA, Phillips SM, Research Group EM: Nutritional regulation of muscle protein synthesis with resistance exercise: strategies to enhance anabolism. Nutr Metab (Lond) 2012;9:40.

13 Tipton, KD, Phillips SM: Dietary protein for muscle hypertrophy; in van Loon LJC, Meeusen R: Limits of Human Endurance. Nestlé Nutr Inst Workshop Ser. Vevey, Nestec/Basel, Karger, 2013, vol 76, pp 73–84.

14 Jeukendrup AE, Chambers ES: Oral carbohydrate sensing and exercise performance. Curr Opin Clin Nutr Metab Care 2010;13:447–451.

15 Burke LM, Hawley JA, Wong SH, Jeukendrup AE: Carbohydrates for training and competition. J Sports Sci 2011;29(suppl 1):S17–S27.

16 Jeukendrup AE: Carbohydrate and exercise performance: the role of multiple transportable carbohydrates. Curr Opin Clin Nutr Metab Care 2010;13:452–457.

17 Cox GR, Clark SA, Cox AJ, Halson SL, Hargreaves M, Hawley JA, Jeacocke N, Snow RJ, Yeo WK, Burke LM: Daily training with high carbohydrate availability increases exogenous carbohydrate oxidation during endurance cycling. J Appl Physiol 2010;109:126–134.

18 Lansley KE, Winyard PG, Fulford J, Vanhatalo A, Bailey SJ, Blackwell JR, DiMenna FJ, Gilchrist M, Benjamin N, Jones AM: Dietary nitrate supplementation reduces the O2 cost of walking and running: a placebo-controlled study. J Appl Physiol 2011;110:591–600.

19 Bescós R, Sureda A, Tur JA, Pons A: The effect of nitric-oxide-related supplements on human performance. Sports Med 2012;42:99–117.

20 Larson-Meyer DE, Willis KS: Vitamin D and athletes. Curr Sports Med Rep 2010;9:220–226.

21 Philp A, Burke LM, Baar K: Altering endogenous carbohydrate availability to support training adaptations; in Maughan RJ, Burke LM (eds): Sports Nutrition: More Than Just Calories – Triggers for Adaptation. Nestlé Nutr Inst Workshop Ser. Vevey, Nestec/Basel, Karger, 2011, vol 69, pp 19–31.

22 Burke LM: Fueling strategies to optimize performance: training high or training low? Scand J Med Sci Sports 2010;20(suppl 2):48–58.

23 Stellingwerff T, Decombaz J, Harris RC, Boesch C: Optimizing human in vivo dosing and delivery of β-alanine supplements for muscle carnosine synthesis. Amino Acids 2012;43:57–65.

24 Harris R, Stellingwerff T: Effect of β-alanine supplementation on high-intensity exercise performance; in van Loon LJC, Meeusen R: Limits of Human Endurance. Nestlé Nutr Inst Workshop Ser. Vevey, Nestec/Basel, Karger, 2013, vol 76, pp 61–71.

25 Burke LM: Caffeine and sports performance. Appl Physiol Nutr Metab 2008;33:1319–1334.

26 Gleeson M, Williams C: Intense exercise training and immune function; in van Loon LJC, Meeusen R: Limits of Human Endurance. Nestlé Nutr Inst Workshop Ser. Vevey, Nestec/Basel, Karger, 2013, vol 76, pp 39–50.

27 Noakes TD: Waterlogged: The Serious Problem of Overhydration in Endurance Sports. Champaign, Human Kinetics, 2012.

van Loon LJC, Meeusen R (eds): Limits of Human Endurance.
Nestlé Nutr Inst Workshop Ser, vol 76, pp 121–125, (DOI: 10.1159/000351344)
Nestec Ltd., Vevey/S. Karger AG., Basel, © 2013

Concluding Remarks: Nutritional Strategies to Increase Performance Capacity

Luc J.C. van Loon[a] · Romain Meeusen[b]

[a]Department of Human Movement Sciences, NUTRIM School for Nutrition, Toxicology and Metabolism, Maastricht University Medical Centre, Maastricht, The Netherlands; [b]Department of Human Physiology and Sports Medicine, Vrije Universiteit Brussel, Brussels, Belgium

A healthy diet, designed to meet the specific demands imposed upon by the individual athlete's training and competition, forms the basis upon which a maximal performance level can be obtained. Most athletes and coaches are well aware that diet and nutritional support should meet nutrient requirements to compensate for the metabolic demands imposed upon by intense exercise training and competition. As a result, nutritional interventions, with or without the use of specifically designed sports nutrition products, are widely applied to extend the limits of human endurance and improve exercise performance capacity. In the 76th Nestlé Nutrition Institute Workshop, a group of expert scientists in the field of nutrition and exercise discussed the ergogenic properties of various nutritional interventions and presented research to show that dietary strategies can be applied to extend the limits of human endurance.

Caffeine, Exercise and the Brain

The first chapter discusses an ergogenic food compound that most of us consume on a daily basis. Caffeine ingestion (3–6 mg per kg bodyweight) has been shown to improve performance during sustained high-intensity endurance type exercise as well as during exhaustive intermittent type exercise activities. Though the debate on the various mechanisms of action continues, there is general consensus that many of the ergogenic benefits of caffeine are attributed to its effects on the brain. Caffeine acts via its antagonism of the adenosine receptor, modulating the dopaminergic and other neurotransmitter systems. Through this neurochemical interaction, caffeine may improve sustained attention, increase vigilance, and reduce symptoms of fatigue. Furthermore, caffeine intake has also been suggested to reduce skeletal muscle pain and force sensation, leading to a reduction in perceived effort during exercise, thereby increasing the motivation to stretch the limits of human endurance.

Carnitine and Fat Oxidation

During moderate-to-high intensity exercise, muscle glycogen represents, from a quantitative perspective, the most important substrate source. As endogenous glycogen stores are relatively small, it has been proposed that increasing fat oxidative capacity can spare muscle glycogen and, as such, improve performance capacity during sustained exercise. Carnitine plays a key role in regulating fat oxidation in skeletal muscle tissue. As muscle free carnitine availability has been identified as a potential factor limiting fat oxidation during high-intensity exercise, it has been suggested that increasing carnitine availability by oral supplementation may increase fat oxidative capacity and improve endurance performance. Preliminary research tends to indicate that greater skeletal muscle carnitine content may increase performance capacity. However, substantial work is required to assess the impact of (prolonged) carnitine supplementation to increase skeletal muscle carnitine content and to confirm whether this can modulate exercise performance capacity.

Hydration during Intense Exercise Training

Maintenance of proper hydration status is a requirement to maintain performance capacity. Though the focus on proper hydration is generally restricted to competition, *Ron Maughan* in his chapter on hydration during intense exercise training explains that sweat loss and fluid replacement may also have important implications in training. Exercise training in the hydrated state and resuming proper hydration immediately after exercise seem more appropriate to support the adaptive response to training than training in a hypohydrated state. Despite the latter, many athletes start their training sessions in a dehydrated state. The most practical way to keep track of changes in the hydration state is to assess changes in bodyweight before and after training sessions. To maintain euhydration, athletes should be taught to increase tolerance to the intake of greater volumes of fluid, especially during prolonged exercise and exercise in the heat, by integrating proper drinking behavior in their training regimen.

Intense Exercise Training and Immune Function

When compared with a sedentary lifestyle, regular moderate-intensity exercise will reduce the risk of infection. However, prolonged bouts of intense exercise and periods of intensified training have been associated with an increased infection risk, particularly when these periods occur in combination with limited recovery time and/or an inadequate energy intake. Effective strategies that can limit immunodepression and minimize the risk of infection include avoidance of people showing early signs of infection and adopting good oral, hand and food hygiene. Furthermore, adequate sleep, reduced psychological stress, no energy intake restriction, and the use of a healthy, balanced diet will reduce the negative impact of intense exercise training on immune function. Finally, nutritional strategies such as carbohydrate provision during prolonged exercise and daily consumption of plant polyphenols and/or *Lactobacillus* probiotics were mentioned as potential effective strategies to attenuate a decline in immune function during intense exercise training and, as such, may help to increase training efficiency and improve performance.

Physiological and Performance Adaptations to High-Intensity Interval Training

High-intensity interval training (HIIT) has recently been advocated as an effective type of exercise training to allow more rapid physiological remodeling when compared with traditional endurance type exercise training. Such HIIT is composed of short bursts of vigorous activity, interspersed by short periods of low-intensity exercise or complete rest. These training sessions are typically short and have been shown to be as effective as more traditional exercise workouts. Consequently, HIIT has been advocated as an efficient intervention strategy to allow more rapid adaptation to exercise training. It has been suggested that HIIT can be used to further improve performance in elite athletes by integrating HIIT into the already high training volume. In this chapter, *Martin Gibala* and *Andrew Jones* speculate that an optimal training intensity distribution for elite endurance athletes should include 10–15% of the training volume composed of exercise at such high exercise intensities.

Effect of β-Alanine Supplementation on High-Intensity Exercise Performance

β-Alanine supplementation increases carnosine levels in skeletal muscle tissue in humans. The greater carnosine levels have been shown to increase exercise capacity and exercise performance in several types of exercise tasks, particularly where the high-intensity exercise range is 1–6 min. Consequently, β-alanine supplementation has become widespread in a variety of athletes to increase endurance in high-intensity track and field, cycling, rowing, swimming events and other competitions.

Dietary Protein for Muscle Hypertrophy

Resistance type exercise stimulates muscle protein synthesis resulting in skeletal muscle hypertrophy. Protein ingestion following exercise increases post-exercise muscle protein synthesis rates, resulting in greater net muscle protein accretion. Though post-exercise muscle protein synthesis rates are generally highest when dietary protein is ingested immediately after exercise, studies have shown that the muscle protein synthetic response to protein ingestion is still increased 24 h after a single bout of exercise. Ingestion of 20–25 g of a high-quality protein is sufficient to maximize post-exercise muscle protein synthesis rates, though more dietary protein may be required in older individuals. Coingestion of large amounts of carbohydrate is not required to maximize the post-exercise muscle protein synthetic response. A healthy diet with smart timing of the dietary protein ingestion after each bout of exercise will augment skeletal muscle hypertrophy during prolonged exercise training and, as such, enhances performance capacity.

The Role of Amino Acids in Skeletal Muscle Adaptation to Exercise

Protein ingestion stimulates muscle protein synthesis. This postprandial muscle protein synthetic response seems to be mainly driven by the essential amino acids, and in particular leucine, that activate the mammalian target of rapamycin. As discussed in the chapter on 'Dietary protein for muscle hypertrophy', protein ingestion following exercise further augments the exercise-driven increase in myofibrillar protein synthesis rate, thereby facilitating skeletal muscle repair and reconditioning. To facilitate the skeletal muscle adaptive response to (resistance type) exercise training, it is advised to ingest 20–25 g of a high-quality protein immediately after exercise. Over the remainder of the day, meals containing 20–25 g protein should be consumed every 4–5 h with a 20–40 g bolus prior to sleep. So far, research data seem to indicate that such a dietary strategy will complement intense exercise training and, as such, support an increase in performance capacity.

National Nutritional Programs for the 2012 London Olympic Games

It has been well established that a healthy balanced diet is required to optimize performance capacity and challenge the limits of human endurance. Specific nutritional interventions as discussed in the previous chapters can further improve performance capacity in specific exercise tasks. In the last chapter, 3 nutritionists responsible for the National Nutrition Programs involved with the 2012 London Olympic Games preparation of the Australian, British and American sports systems express their challenges to ensure proper diet and effective nutritional interventions for the Olympic athletes from the viewpoints of the Australian Institute of Sport, the English Institute of Sport and the United States Olympic Committee.

The aim of this workshop was to explore some of the properties of various nutritional interventions to improve exercise performance capacity and, as such, to extend the limits of human endurance. This book summarizes the work that was discussed during the workshop, and we hope it has provided the reader with novel insights into the complex interaction between nutrition and exercise, allowing him/her to define more effective dietary strategies to improve health and performance.

Subject Index

Adenosine, caffeine effects in brain 2–4, 10, 122
β-Alanine, *see also* M-Carn
    carnosine synthesis 64
    M-Carn formation and muscle effects 61, 62, 64, 65
    supplementation effects 64–69, 124
Allergy, upper respiratory tract infection association 47
Amino acids, *see* Protein, dietary
Attention, caffeine effects in brain 5, 6

B cell, intensive training effects 41, 42

Caffeine
    brain modulation
        adenosine 2–4, 10, 122
        attention 5, 6
        dopamine 3, 4, 6, 11
        fatigue reduction 5, 6
        motor drive 3, 4, 7, 8
    muscle effects
        fatigue reduction 6, 7
        pain reduction 6
        perceived effort 7
        tremor 8
    overview of effects 1, 2
    placebo effects in exercise performance 8–10
    temperature effects on exercise performance response 10
Carbohydrate
    protein coingestion effects 81, 82, 97

uptake and water balance 32
Carnitine
    cycle in fat oxidation 14–16
    fat oxidation
        functional overview 14–16
        regulation in muscle
            availability effects 19, 20
            endurance performance response 21
            role 18, 19, 122
    palmitoyltransferase 14–18
Carnosine, *see* M-Carn

Dehydration, *see* Water balance
Dopamine, caffeine effects in brain 3, 4, 6, 11

Elongation factor 2 kinase (eEF2K), mTOR regulation 87, 88
Essential amino acids, *see* Protein, dietary

Fatigue, caffeine reduction 5–7
Fat oxidation
    carnitine role 14–16, 122
    regulation in muscle
        carnitine
            availability effects 19, 20
            endurance performance response 21
            role 18, 19
        rate 16–18
4E-BP1, mTOR regulation 87

Glycogen, depletion delay by fat
oxidation 13, 14

High-intensity interval training (HIIT)
adaptation to low-volume training in
recreation and untrained
individuals 52–55, 59
overview 51, 52
performance improvement in highly
trained individuals 55–59, 123
Hydration, *see* Water balance

Immune response
amino acid effects after intense
exercise 91–93
guidelines for maintenance in
athletes 43–48
infection transmission prevention
45
intensive training and
depression 41–43, 123
upper respiratory tract infection in
athletes 40, 41, 48
Infection, *see* Immune response

LAT1, mTOR activation role 90, 93
Leucine, uptake and mTOR
activation 89–91

Maximal oxygen uptake (VO$_{2max}$), high
intensity interval training adaptation
studies 52–56
M-Carn, *see also* β-Alanine
acid buffering in muscle 62, 63
calcium ion sensitivity effects 63
ergogenic effects
long-duration submaximal exercise
performance 66–69
maximal/supramaximal exercise
performance 66
overview 65, 66
glycation 63
synthesis from β-alanine 61, 62, 64,
65
Motor drive, caffeine effects in brain 3, 4,
7, 8
mTOR

activation
exercise 86, 87
leucine uptake role 89–91
mechanisms 88, 89
functional overview 87, 88
protein supplementation and
endurance adaptation 91
Muscle
caffeine effects, *see* Caffeine
fat oxidation, *see* Fat oxidation
hypertrophy, *see* Protein, dietary
mTOR regulation, *see* mTOR

National sports nutrition program
Australia 104, 115
clinical nutrition needs of
athletes 109, 110
food service at London
Olympics 111–114
Great Britain 104, 116
implementation of updated
knowledge 104–108
outcomes review after London
Olympics 115–119, 125
Ramadan nutrition challenges at
London Olympics 111
special nutrition services at London
Olympics 114, 115
systems development 105, 108, 109
United States 104, 116
Nutrition program, *see* National sports
nutrition program

Olympics, *see* National sports nutrition
program

Pain, caffeine in reduction 6
Peak power output (PPO), high-intensity
interval training effects 57
Potassium, sweat loss 29, 30
Protein, dietary
essential amino acids and muscle
protein synthesis 86
muscle hypertrophy studies
amount of protein 78, 79, 94, 95
carbohydrate coingestion
effects 81, 82, 97

fat coingestion effects 81
inactivity studies 81, 82
metabolic basis 74
methodology 74, 75
muscle protein breakdown 74, 75, 78
muscle protein synthesis 74–81
net muscle protein balance 74–77, 79, 81
protein type and anabolic response 76, 77, 96, 97
timing of ingestion 79, 80, 95, 96
supplementation
amino acid attenuation of exercise-induced immunosuppression 91–93
endurance adaptation 91
practical guidelines 93, 94, 98, 124, 125

RagD, mTOR activation role 88, 89
Ramadan, nutrition challenges at London Olympics 111
Rheb, mTOR activation role 8

S6K1, mTOR regulation 87, 88
SNAT2, mTOR activation role 90
Sodium, balance in exercise 29, 30

Splanchic blood flow (SBF), exercise response 31
Sports nutrition program, see National sports nutrition program

T cell, intensive training effects 41–43
T cell receptor excision circle (TREC) 43
Tremor, caffeine induction 8

Upper respiratory tract infection (URTI)
allergy association 47
risks and management in athletes 40, 41, 48

Water balance
beverage temperature effects 32, 33
dehydration adaptation and coping 33
gut training 32, 33
hydration and training response 33–35, 122, 123
overview of optimization for exercise performance 25–27, 35
rehydration and recovery between training bouts 31, 32
stress response 30, 31
turnover measurement in sports 27–29